Adult
Physical Disabilities
Case Studies for Learning

Adult
Physical Disabilities
Case Studies for Learning

Lori T. Andersen, EdD, OTR/L
Florida International University
Miami, Florida

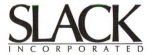

SLACK
INCORPORATED

An innovative information, education and management company
6900 Grove Road • Thorofare, NJ 08086

Copyright © 2002 by SLACK Incorporated

All rights reserved. No part of this book may be reproduced, stored in a retrieval system or transmitted in any form or by any means, electronic, mechanical, photocopying, recording or otherwise, without written permission from the publisher, except for brief quotations embodied in critical articles and reviews.

The procedures and practices described in this book should be implemented in a manner consistent with the professional standards set for the circumstances that apply in each specific situation. Every effort has been made to confirm the accuracy of the information presented and to correctly relate generally accepted practices. The author, editor, and publisher cannot accept responsibility for errors or exclusions or for the outcome of the application of the material presented herein. There is no expressed or implied warranty of this book or information imparted by it.

The work SLACK publishes is peer reviewed. Prior to publication, recognized leaders in the field, educators, and clinicians provide important feedback on the concepts and content that we publish. We welcome feedback on this work.

Printed in the United States of America.

Andersen, Lori T.
  Adult physical disabilities : case studies for learning / Lori T. Andersen.
    p. ; cm
Includes bibliographical references and index.
  ISBN 1-55642-537-6 (alk. paper)
1. Medical rehabilitation--Case studies.
  [DNLM: 1. Rehabilitation--Aged--Case Report. 2. Geriatric Assessment--Case Report. 3. Musculoskeletal System--physiopathology--Aged--Case Report. 4. Occupational Therapy--methods--Case Report. 5. Physical Therapy--Aged--Case Report. WB 460 A544a 2001] I. Title.
  RM930.A553 2001
  617'.03--dc21

                          2001049633

Published by: SLACK Incorporated
                6900 Grove Road
                Thorofare, NJ 08086 USA
                Telephone: 856-848-1000
                Fax: 856-853-5991
                www.slackbooks.com

Contact SLACK Incorporated for more information about other books in this field or about the availability of our books from distributors outside the United States.

Authorization to photocopy items for internal or personal use, or the internal or personal use of specific clients, is granted by SLACK Incorporated, provided that the appropriate fee is paid directly to Copyright Clearance Center, 222 Rosewood Drive, Danvers, MA 01923 USA, 978-750-8400. Prior to photocopying items for educational classroom use, please contact the CCC at the address above. Please reference Account Number 9106324 for SLACK Incorporated's Professional Book Division.

For further information on CCC, check CCC Online at the following address: http://www.copyright.com.

Last digit is print number: 10   9   8   7   6   5   4   3   2   1

DEDICATION

To all past, present, and future students

CONTENTS

Instructors: *Adult Physical Disabilities: Case Studies for Learning Instructor's Manual* is also available from SLACK Incorporated. Don't miss this important companion to *Adult Physical Disabilities: Case Studies for Learning* available at http://www.efacultylounge.com.

ACKNOWLEDGMENTS

First, I wish to acknowledge and thank Barbara L. Kornblau, JD, OTR/L, FAOTA, DAAPM, ABDA, CDMS, CCM, who in her unique way, helped me to go beyond myself and accomplish things I never thought possible. I am deeply indebted to my colleagues, Carol Niman Reed, EdD, OTR/L, FAOTA and Sandee Dunbar, MA, OTR/L for their sharing and caring, as together we learned about this case-based method. Also, many thanks to Karen Berry Ayala, MS, OTR/L and Cheryl Acheson Reed, MS, OTR/L, CHT who graciously contributed case studies for this book. And finally, my gratitude is extended to the Charter Class (1997) at Nova Southeastern University for helping me to learn, and for their appreciation of this educational method.

ABOUT THE AUTHOR

Lori T. Andersen, EdD, OTR/L received her bachelor's degree from Springfield College, Massachusetts, her master's degree in Occupational Therapy from the Medical College of Virginia, and her doctoral degree from Nova Southeastern University, Ft. Lauderdale, Florida. Entering academia in 1994, she has served on the faculties at Florida International University in Miami, Florida and Nova Southeastern University. Prior to her career in academia, she worked in clinical practice in a variety of settings including acute care, home health, and rehabilitation. She has also served as chairperson of the Florida Occupational Therapy Council (licensure body) and vice president of the Florida Occupational Therapy Association. In her spare time she enjoys traveling, antiquing, and furniture refinishing.

CONTRIBUTING AUTHORS

Karen Berry Ayala, MS, OTR/L received her bachelor's degree in psychology from Radford University, Virginia and her master's degree in Occupational Therapy from Boston University, Massachusetts. Karen has a diverse background in Occupational Therapy. She has worked as a staff therapist at the Miami VA Medical Center, instructor of OT at Nova Southeastern University in Fort Lauderdale, FL, and lead hand therapist and ergonomic consultant at a private hand therapy clinic in El Cerrito, CA. Currently, Karen is a senior hand therapist and ergonomic consultant with NovaCare Outpatient Rehabilitation in Hayward, CA. In her spare time, Karen enjoys running marathons and traveling.

Barbara L. Kornblau, JD, OTR/L, FAOTA, DAAPM, ABDA, CDMS, CCM is an OT and practicing attorney. A graduate of the University of Wisconsin-Madison and the University of Miami School of Law, she has lectured internationally and published extensively on medicolegal issues. She has served in many volunteer roles for AOTA including President of the AOTA (2001-2003). She is a member of the faculty of Nova Southeastern University and is the mother of six children. Her occupations include reading, quilting, genealogy, and serving the community through the South Miami Rotary Club.

Cheryl Acheson Reed, MS, OTR/L, CHT received her bachelor of science degree in Occupational Therapy from Eastern Michigan University and her master of science in Occupational Therapy from Wayne State University, Detroit, MI. She has had experience in a variety of therapeutic settings, with a concentration in hand therapy. She has been an adjunct professor at several universities in Michigan and Florida, teaching subjects such as hand/upper extremity therapy, kinesiology, and conditions. She also owns and operates the Southern Palm Bed & Breakfast in Loxahatchee, Florida.

PREFACE

This workbook is designed to foster student learning about adult rehabilitation and to develop clinical reasoning. The workbook contains 35 case studies about various clients with orthopedic injuries, rheumatic disease, amputations, spinal cord injuries, hand injuries, burns, strokes, brain injuries, multiple sclerosis, as well as clients who are injured workers, or workers at risk. This case-based approach actively engages students in solving the problem of developing an effective evaluation and treatment plan for various clients. These case studies describe clients and situations one may encounter in practice, making learning more relevant to actual practice, helping students make that transition from the classroom to the clinic. Case study worksheets provide a structure and format for students to "think aloud" as they develop treatment planning and documentation skills. Occupational therapy instructors will find this workbook to be a valuable course tool as it offers a structured process and a framework through which students learn treatment planning skills, linking theory to practice.

This workbook is a product of a case-based educational approach used to teach Master's level occupational therapy students at Nova Southeastern University, Ft. Lauderdale, Florida. In this course, Occupational Therapy in Physical Disabilities and Work Practice, students worked in small groups to learn treatment planning. The objective was for students to develop clinical reasoning, self-directed learning, and lifelong learning skills. These are the skills necessary to continue to develop beyond entry-level practice and to maintain competence in an era of continual advancement of knowledge and technology and the ever-changing health care arena.

Chapters 1 and 2 describe the step-by-step process used in this case-based approach and the students' or group members' roles in this process. Chapter 3 provides a step-by-step example of the process students use to "solve" a case study problem and develop a treatment plan. Completed example worksheets are included in Chapter 3.

Chapters 4 through 10 are three part case studies. The three parts simulate the thought process and treatment planning process from when a referral is received (Part 1), to determining which assessments and assessment tools are most appropriate (Part 2), to developing a treatment plan based on the evaluation data (Part 3). Chapters 11 through 37 are case studies that provide evaluation data in one part, requiring students to develop a treatment plan only. The case studies are sequenced from "simpler" orthopedic cases to "more difficult" neurological cases. However, when proceeding through the sequence, having learned the step-by-step process of treatment planning used in this workbook, the later case study problems become easier rather than more difficult to solve. Emphasis in this workbook focuses on developing treatment plans that are occupation-based and client-centered. Activity analysis is also emphasized as students must specifically describe and grade activities to be used in treatment.

My wish is that all students who use this workbook enjoy this collaborative learning process, as they become skilled practitioners. Additionally, I hope they see the benefit of this educational method for developing self-directed and life long learning skills to remain competent in practice.

FOREWORD

Thomas Edison very keenly stated, "Thinking is hard work." *Adult Physical Disabilities: Case Studies for Learning* by Lori T. Andersen is a tool developed to help occupational therapy students and practitioners with the process of thinking as it applies to occupational therapy clinical practice. Her case studies foster creative and insightful thinking in occupational therapy for both students and practitioners. The case studies contained in this book develop thinking skills for problem solving, as well as creative therapeutic intervention to best meet the needs of those we serve while "thinking like an occupational therapy practitioner." This book seeks to make critical, clinical thinking an integral part of one's professional self and not such "hard work."

With this book as a tool, students and practitioners have a springboard from which to develop their own repertoire of treatment interventions and creative ideas. They can move away from cones and pegs and infuse occupation back into practice. As Sydney J. Harris said, "The real danger is not that machines will begin to think like men, but that men will begin to think like machines." This book provides a mechanism to keep students and practitioners thinking creatively and innovatively.

Barbara L. Kornblau, JD, OTR/L, FAOTA, DAAPM, ABDA, CDMS, CCM

1

Case-Based Learning Approach

Give me a fish and I eat for today.
Teach me to fish and I will eat for a lifetime.

Chinese Proverb

INTRODUCTION

The information age, advances in scientific knowledge, new technology, and continual changes in health care delivery systems; all of these require health care practitioners to make an extra effort to remain current in their fields. Early on, students must become self-directed, lifelong learners who are able to take charge of their own learning to continue to acquire knowledge throughout their professional careers. This workbook offers a case-based learning approach designed to help students develop this skill along with clinical-reasoning skills, in order to be effective health care practitioners.

This case-based learning approach is student-centered instead of teacher-centered. In a teacher-centered format, the learning needs of the students are generally determined by the teacher. Students are usually passive participants in learning (i.e., listening to lectures developed by the teacher). In a student-centered format, students determine their own learning needs and develop plans to meet those needs. Students are active participants in the learning process as they gather, share, and evaluate information in the process of solving a case study problem. In solving these problems, students gain knowledge and information that can be used to solve future problems they may encounter.

If you think about it, this problem-solving method is a very common way in which we learn. Think of a hobby that you have. Perhaps that hobby is photography, stamp or coin collecting, trading cards, cooking, sewing, car or motorcycle racing, genealogy, sailing, or other. Your interest in this hobby prompted you in some fashion to develop a plan to learn more about the hobby. Think of the various resources you used to learn your hobby—perhaps books, journal or newspaper articles, or other experts in the field. As you learned, you identified more learning issues and further developed a plan to learn more in-depth.

The process to develop clinical competence is similar. The students learn how to solve case study problems by using their existing knowledge from previous courses and experiences, by defining learning issues (or what they need to learn), by researching the learning issues, and then by using all this information to solve a case study problem. The instructors, in this context called the tutors, guide the students through the process of solving the problem by developing a treatment plan for a specific client.

This case-based learning approach is relevant to actual practice because it simulates the clinical setting using a variety of case studies. In the clinic, the student will encounter a variety of clients with multiple problems. The context of each case will be different. Each client will be a different age, have different cognitive and educational levels, come from a different culture, have different social support systems, have different resources, and have different goals. In developing a treatment plan, the student will need to be able to take all this information into consideration, as well as information about the clinical diagnoses, medical history, prognosis, precautions, and funding sources.

Additionally, as health care practitioners work in teams, it is necessary to learn how to work effectively in a group and how to be a contributing team member. In this case-based learning approach, students learn about the group process and learn how to effectively work in a group for the benefit of the client.

Students previously involved in this method of learning have emphasized the benefit in helping with the transition to the clinic. When evaluating this case-based learning approach, students have made the following comments:

- "I have gained a sense of self-confidence because of this method. I get lost during lectures, but being involved in a group keeps me interested, focused, and requires me to think. I seem to be remembering things much easier."
- "This prepared me for my clinical internship. I was able to research my client's situation and establish an appropriate and effective treatment plan in a reasonable time."
- "This encourages student growth, confidence in ideas, and an increase in professional attitude."

Student supervisors have also written about the ability of the students:

- "Students took initiative to find needed information and used department resources to solve problems."
- "Students demonstrated good analytical skills."

THE TUTORIAL GROUP PROCESS

In the case-based learning approach, one of the main formats used is the tutorial group. A tutorial group usually consists of five to ten students. The students in each group collaborate on developing occupational therapy treatment plans for clients described in assigned case studies. The case study may take any of the following forms: written or paper case study, videotape case study, a simulated (role playing) case study, or a live case study. The cases in this book are written case studies. The group may spend several sessions working on a case study.

Barrows (1994, pp. 49-79) describes the basic sequence of the tutorial group process:

1. The tutorial group is given a case study problem.
2. The tutorial group determines learning issues.
3. The tutorial group members research learning issues.
4. The tutorial group members share their researched information.
5. The tutorial group applies the information to the case study problem.

6. The tutorial group evaluates the resources used.
7. The tutorial group members assess participation and performance of themselves and their peers.

Some of these tasks and steps are ongoing throughout the tutorial group sessions. The tutorial group will be determining learning issues, researching learning issues, sharing information, evaluating resources, and assessing group member participation on an ongoing basis in the collaborative effort to develop a treatment plan. The following are descriptions of the tasks of the tutorial group.

Learning Issues

A learning issue is identified when the members of the group lack the knowledge to solve a problem or to understand a particular concept about the case study. These learning issues, or learning needs, identify the weaknesses in the person's or group's knowledge. While no one likes to acknowledge weaknesses or expose weaknesses to others, it is critical for the health care professional to be able to identify learning issues or needs. Having the skill to identify learning needs and develop and follow a plan to learn will help people to continually learn and improve their level of competence.

Researching Learning Issues

At the end of each session, the group should look at the list of learning issues they generated, group issues by theme, and delegate responsibility for each learning issue to a specific group member. Some learning issues may be assigned to more than one group member. The group member is then responsible to thoroughly research his or her assigned learning issue, and present this information to the group. The group member should document which resources were used. He or she may also want to outline pertinent information about the case study problem and learning issue for copying and distribution to the tutorial group and other class members. For overall learning, it would be very beneficial for each group member to do research, at least superficially, on all the identified learning issues. This will facilitate each group member's participation in the tutorial sessions and will help each group member to learn the course material.

Finding Resources

There are a variety of resources that can be used for developing treatment plans for the case studies. The required and recommended course textbooks are valuable resources. The table of contents in textbooks is perhaps the most obvious place to look to find out where to locate information about a specific topic. The index of the textbook is instrumental in looking up where key words or key phrases are located. Usually a bibliography or reference list is found at the end of each chapter or at the end of the book. These reference listings of other books and articles may also be pertinent for research on your learning issue. Many of these books or articles may be found in your university library or can be obtained by interlibrary loan.

Your textbooks will be helpful, but by no means should they be the only resource used. The university library will have many books and professional journals that will be useful for researching information. The library computers can be used to find appropriate books, professional journals, and specific journal articles. Again, if materials are not available in the university library, interlibrary loan services may be able to obtain this information for you. The librarian will be most willing to help you to use any of the library resources.

With the advances in technology, the Internet can be used to find pertinent information and a variety of resources. Other resources to consider are professors, health care professionals in the community, guest speakers who have presented in your classes, and even your fellow students who have experience in certain areas. These personal resources are usually flattered that you have sought them out as long as you make sure that you have contacted them at a convenient time. Please remember to thank them for their assistance.

Sharing Information

Sharing of information will take place in many ways because the case-based learning method emphasizes cooperative and collaborative learning.

First, sharing of information will take place during tutorial group sessions which focus on "brainstorming" and discussion of those ideas. Remember that when brainstorming, everyone is encouraged to generate ideas and all ideas are considered without judgment or comments from others. You will have structured questions and formatted worksheets that will help to guide the group in problem-solving.

In these sessions, a person should be designated as the recorder. The role of recorder should be rotated so that everyone gets a chance to record results of the group discussions. The formatted worksheet can easily be copied on the whiteboard or blackboard and "filled in" as the group discussion progresses. It is strongly suggested that the recorder write on a whiteboard or blackboard for all group members to see what has been discussed so far. As the group discussion progresses, if the group decides to change their ideas, it is very easy to edit the worksheet.

Another group member should copy the information from the board to a paper copy of the formatted worksheet. These papers can then be copied for distribution to all group members. Time will be wasted if all group members try to take all their own notes on the group discussion.

Second, information on the researched learning issues will be shared at various tutorial group sessions. This sharing of information may take the form of written communication, including reference lists, outlines, and summaries of material researched. Researched information can also be shared verbally in the tutorial sessions. All group members are encouraged to ask questions during the tutorial sessions to clarify information. Group members should not take offense at questions. Questioning is one way in which we learn. Questions frequently help all group members to understand the material better. Questions also help the person answering the question to learn to express him or herself better verbally.

Through both of these methods of sharing information, the student will develop written and verbal communication skills.

Applying Information to the Case Study Problem

Once tutorial group members have researched learning issues and have shared this information, the tutorial group must critically analyze the information to determine if it is relevant to the case study problem. In applying the information to the case study problem, tutorial group members should ask such questions as:

1. What does the information mean in relation to the case?
2. Is the information helpful and appropriate in view of the client diagnosis, prognosis, precautions, resources, and discharge plans?

In applying the information to the case study problem, group members need to explain their rationale and justify their choice of treatment approach, technique, or strategy using valid resources.

Evaluating Resources

In the tutorial group session, each group member should evaluate the resources that were used to find information about the learning issue. Some factors that need to be taken into consideration in evaluating a resource include:

1. Was the resource difficult to find?
2. Was the information from a peer reviewed resource?
3. How recent was the resource? Was the information outdated?

4. Is the information given by the resource reliable and valid?
5. Was the resource too simplistic and superficial?
6. Did the resource give comprehensive and detailed information about the learning issue?
7. Was the resource difficult to understand?

Sometimes various resources will contradict each other. Keep in mind that often there are different opinions and appropriate ways to accomplish the same goal.

It is important to be able to evaluate resources to determine what information, if any, should be used. Also, knowing which resources were more beneficial will generally save time the next time resources need to be sought out.

Peer- and Self-Assessments

The skill to assess abilities and learning needs is an essential skill for self-directed, lifelong learning. This skill is needed in order to remain effective and contemporary in practice. The ability to provide constructive feedback to peers is also a necessary skill for a person to be an effective member of a health care team (Barrows, 1994, p. 30; Hay, 1995).

All group members will evaluate themselves and their peers on their effectiveness as collaborative group members, their ability to determine learning issues and needs, their ability to find pertinent resources, and their ability to critically analyze and synthesize information. It is each group member's responsibility to provide honest and constructive feedback to other group members on their performance in the tutorial sessions and to be honest, critical, and constructive in evaluating his or her own performance as well. Comparing the self-assessment to the peer-assessment will help group members to see how his or her self-perception of his or her participation compares to how others perceive his or her participation. Using self-assessment, constructive feedback, and comparisons of peer- and self-assessments will assist group members to improve his or her self-assessment skills, as well as to improve his or her performance. This will help the group members grow as a professionals and self-directed, lifelong learners.

Peer- and self-assessment forms may potentially be completed at the end of each tutorial session, at the end of the case study, at midterm, and/or at the end of the course. An example of the peer and self-assessment form is provided in Table 1-1.

Students may wish to see an actual tutorial group session to more fully understand the process. *The Tutorial Process in Problem-Based Learning* developed by Barrows and MacRae (1992), is an excellent video recording of a tutorial group session. In this video recording, the tutorial group, composed of medical students at Southern Illinois University, uses the tutorial group process to solve a case study problem.

Table 1-1

Peer- and Self-Assessment

Name of person being assessed_____

Evaluator's name_____

Indicate level of agreement for each statement using this five point scale:

Strongly				**Strongly**
Disagree	**Disagree**	**Neutral**	**Agree**	**Agree**
1	2	3	4	5

1. Degree of respect for/responsibility to group

    ___You/they attended and participated in all group sessions.

    ___You/they were prompt in attendance.

    ___You/they followed through on assignments made by the group.

    ___You/they were flexible and available for scheduling of additional group sessions
      when needed.

    ___You/they listened to and facilitated other points of view.

Comments:

2. Contribution to the group process

    ___You/they made positive contributions to the group process.

    ___You/they encouraged others to participate.

    ___You/they helped keep the group on task and focused.

    ___You/they facilitated group problem-solving.

Comments:

3. Ability to determine learning needs

    ___You/they contributed to defining the learning issues.

    ___You/they were able to determine what needed to be learned in order to facilitate solving
      the problem.

Comments:

4. Ability to find resources and contribute information to the group

    ___The information you/they contributed was relative to the problem.

    ___You/they were able to find appropriate and contemporary resources.

    ___You/they sought a variety of resources.

Comments:

5. Ability to critically analyze and synthesize information

    ___You/they critically reviewed information for accuracy and pertinence.

    ___You/they were able to explain difficult information to the group.

    ___You/they related the information to the specific case incorporating a client-centered approach.

    ___You/they were able to judge what information is pertinent to the case and what is not, based on
      the uniqueness of the specific case.

Total_____

The Tutorial Group

GROUP MEMBER RESPONSIBILITIES

Adults prefer to learn in comfortable learning situations. To create a comfortable learning situation for all, it is important for all group members to show respect for everyone in class. Everyone has their own opinions, and everyone makes mistakes and errors. It is important to show tolerance for different opinions and for the mistakes and errors of yourself and others.

The students have certain responsibilities to the group in this collaborative learning effort for the group to be effective. All students are responsible for attending each group session, to come on time to each group session, and to be prepared for each group session. All students are responsible for participating actively in each session and also for facilitating each group member's participation and opinion. All group members are also responsible for giving positive and constructive feedback to their colleagues during the tutorial sessions. This feedback will help everyone to learn and to grow as a clinician.

ROLE OF THE TUTOR

The tutor helps to facilitate the tutorial group process and to guide student learning. This is done by asking probing questions to help the group members use their existing knowledge and develop learning issues and needs. Responsibilities of the tutor include encouraging student participation, ensuring all group members participate, helping the group members evaluate their learning and assess their effectiveness as group members, and giving constructive feedback. The tutor is not responsible for giving students information, but rather to help the students discover specific content areas and analyze information through probing questions. The main objective of the tutor is to develop all group members into independent learners. Therefore, the tutor encourages discussion and questioning among group members and gradually withdraws from participating in the group.

GROUP MEMBER ROLES

For efficient group functioning, a variety of roles need to be assumed by the group members. The role of the tutor is preassigned to the instructors. In normal groups, certain task roles and group maintenance roles are voluntarily taken by the members of the group. These roles help the group to meet its objectives and maintain group cohesiveness. If the group becomes bogged down, the members should look to see if it is because members may not be demonstrating characteristics or behaviors of the various task and group maintenance roles. Nonfunctional group roles interfere with the group process. When a student demonstrates the characteristics or behaviors of a nonfunctional group role, the group needs to identify and deal with the problem.

Task Roles

Each tutorial group has a task or objective to achieve in developing a treatment plan for a particular client in the case study. Various task roles are often taken by group members to help the group accomplish their goal. These roles are generally not assigned. A person may hold or demonstrate the characteristics and behaviors of more than one of these task roles. Mosey (1976, p. 46) and Borg and Bruce (1991, p. 113) have described various task roles. These task roles are:

- Initiator-contributor: This person gives suggestions and ideas to provide direction to the group to help accomplish the task.
- Information seeker: This person asks questions to help obtain the needed information or to clarify information.
- Information giver: This person gives information based on facts that have been researched and/or from personal experiences.
- Opinion seeker: This person asks questions to get clarification of opinions and values.
- Opinion giver: This person gives personal opinions and values and/or gives other opinions and values for the group to consider.
- Elaborator: This person explains information and suggestions made by other group members in more detail.
- Coordinator: This person suggests relationships between ideas and concepts. This person also attempts to coordinate group activities.
- Orienter: This person sums up the position of the group in order to help the group set a future course or plan of action.
- Evaluator: This person evaluates progress and accomplishments of the group.
- Energizer: This person stimulates the group to take such actions as brainstorming and presenting ideas and making decisions about how to proceed with the task at hand.
- Procedural technician: This person assists the group by performing routine tasks such as copying written materials.
- Recorder: This person acts as the group secretary. As stated earlier, this role should be rotated among group members.

Group Maintenance Roles

Borg and Bruce (1991, p. 114) and Mosey (1976, p. 47) also describe social-emotional roles or group maintenance roles that help group function by meeting members' needs. Again these roles are not assigned and group members may demonstrate the behaviors of more than one of these roles. These group maintenance or social-emotional roles are:

- Encourager: This person gives positive feedback to group members and acknowledges and accepts their contributions to the group.
- Harmonizer: This person mediates group conflicts and helps to reduce tension in the group.
- Compromiser: This person will modify his or her position and put aside personal needs for the benefit of the group.
- Gatekeeper: This person facilitates communication and encourages equal participation for all group members by preventing one or two people from monopolizing the group.
- Standard setter: This person reminds the group of protocol, how group members should act, and group standards and values.
- Observer: This person monitors the group's activities and gives feedback about group performance.
- Follower: This person is a passive participant who accepts group decisions and does not interfere with the group process.

Nonfunctional Group Roles

Hill (1977, p. 38) and Borg and Bruce (1991, p. 115) describe nonfunctional group member roles. These roles or behaviors exhibited in these roles interfere with the group process. Group members may demonstrate the behaviors of more than one of these roles. These roles exhibited are:

- Aggressor: This person may use malicious and sarcastic humor, attacks others' ideas, or may take credit inappropriately.
- Blocker: This person interferes with the group's progress by continually arguing points, refusing to consider ideas, or going off on tangents.
- Recognition seeker: This person prevents group progress by continuously seeking attention and/or projecting a superior attitude.
- Self-confessor: This person continually discusses personal concerns and/or individual agendas rather than the group's agenda.
- "Horse player": This person derails group progress through lazy attitude and nonproductive activity such as excessive joking.
- Sympathy seeker: This person continually seeks attention and pity by expressing personal insecurities.

- Special interest pleader: This person continually promotes personal biases and prejudices on the pretense of speaking for others.
- Dominator: This person intentionally controls and manipulates others.
- Withdrawer: This person interferes with group progress by not taking responsibility as a group member to actively participate in the group process.
- Competitor: This person interferes with the group progress by always trying to do better than others rather than collaborating with group members for the benefit of all.

GROUP DYNAMICS

According to Borg and Bruce (1991, p. 108), there are four phases of group development. First, as the group is forming, the group members are learning about each other as well as the purpose of the group. At this stage, the group members can learn about the backgrounds their colleagues have had in occupational therapy or related fields. It is helpful to know this so that the group members can act as resource people for various case studies. In the second phase, as the group members get to know each other, personality conflicts may develop. As the group deals with resolving these conflicts they move into the third stage where the conflict diminishes and the group becomes more cohesive. Finally, the group will hit their stride and the group process will become more productive. The group will be able to see its successes and appreciate the benefit in working together collaboratively.

Working in a group does not always go smoothly. Group members have different personalities, learning styles, and schedules. Inherent in this is the potential for arguments and conflicts about how the group should be run and when group sessions should take place. It is not unusual for the group to run into some problems with group dynamics. Some disagreement and conflict can be healthy for the group. People have different opinions and different ways of solving problems. Differing opinions can help the group to see different viewpoints and improve the effectiveness of the treatment plans that are developed. However, groups might see some of the nonfunctional group roles and behaviors emerging. These behaviors throw the group off task. When this occurs, it is important for the group to recognize and deal with some of these issues in order to resolve the conflicts so that the group may get back to the task of developing a treatment plan for the client. Being able to work effectively in groups is important because students will most likely be working as a member of a health care team.

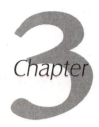

Chapter

Case Study Example

Occupational therapy students, when confronted with their first client, often have that panicked look and response, "What do I do?" The student should take a deep breath and then take the time to think about and proceed through the problem-solving process of developing a treatment or intervention plan. This chapter provides an example of the problem-solving or clinical reasoning process of developing a treatment or intervention plan. For purposes of this book, the treatment or intervention plan will be referred to as the treatment plan.

In occupational therapy, the clinical reasoning process includes five types of processes described by Fleming (1991), Neistadt (1998), Neistadt, Wight, and Mulligan (1998), and Mattingly and Fleming (1994). The five types of reasoning processes are listed below:

1. *Procedural reasoning* focuses on the client's injury, illness, or disease and the resulting functional limitations.

2. *Narrative reasoning* focuses on the roles, tasks, and activities that are valued by the client.

3. *Interactive reasoning* focuses on the client's perception of the injury, illness, or disease and the meaning it has for the client.

4. *Pragmatic reasoning* focuses on the current treatment environment and resources available, including physical, social, and financial resources as well as skills of the treating therapist(s).

5. *Conditional reasoning* focuses on the planning needed to enable the client to function in a future situation or environment such as discharge environment.

These reasoning processes are used to develop a client-centered treatment plan that is effective and efficient. In a client-centered approach, the occupational therapist collaborates closely with the client in developing and implementing a treatment plan. As each client is unique and is in the best position to know which occupations are meaningful to him or her, the occupational therapist draws on the knowledge and experience of the client, making him or her an active participant in the therapy process (Law, Polatajko, Baptiste, & Townsend, 1997).

As a student, you are still learning, so the clinical reasoning process will take more time. As you gain experience, you will move through the process faster as you formulate questions and answers almost instantaneously, without perceiving that you have done so. Even the most experienced therapist does not always know exactly what to do when first assigned a case. Experienced therapists determine the treatment plan through data gathering, including interviews with clients and significant others, assessments, consultations with team members and other health care professionals, and through the use of other resources. Follow the process and the treatment plan will unfold. The case study in this chapter provides an example of this process.

IDENTIFYING LEARNING ISSUES

Part 1

Maggie is a 61-year-old female referred to home health occupational therapy on October 29 with a diagnosis of right Colles fracture. Maggie fell while shopping at her neighborhood department store on October 27. The physician has ordered occupational therapy to evaluate and treat.

Analysis of Part 1

Often times the occupational therapist will be given the client's name and diagnosis and little else. The information given above is typical of the information you may be given to start a case. With this information the therapist can start to think about how the case should be approached. Even though the information given is minimal, there is much that you probably already know about the case. Think about what you know already and what you will need to know to effectively manage the case. You may have learned this information from school and/or from life experiences.

For example: (Type of reasoning is indicated in parentheses)

- Do you know what a Colles fracture is? (procedural reasoning)
- Do you know what the clinical signs and symptoms of a Colles fracture are? Complicating factors? (procedural reasoning)
- Do you know the medical management for a Colles fracture? Precautions? (procedural reasoning)
- What is the prognosis of recovery post Colles fracture? (procedural reasoning)
- What might this woman "look like" and be able to do 2 days post Colles fracture? (procedural reasoning)
- Do you have an image of the capabilities of a 61-year-old woman who goes shopping? (narrative reasoning)
- Might this image give you some indication of her prior level of function and roles as well as an idea of her discharge situation and goals? (conditional reasoning)

Answer the following questions on the Tutorial Session Sheet (Figure 3-1a). At this point, your questions and plan need not focus on specifics of evaluation (e.g., range of motion [ROM] will be assessed using a goniometer) of Maggie because evaluation will be addressed in Part 2 of the case study.

Questions: Part 1

1. What do you already know that will help you to approach this case? What knowledge has prepared you to approach this case? What do you know about:
   a) Individual client—roles, tasks, activities
   b) The client's physical/sociocultural environment
   c) Clinical signs and symptoms, treatment for diagnosis
2. What questions do you have that need to be answered to effectively manage this case? What do you need to learn? What do you need to learn about:
   a) Individual client—roles, tasks, activities
   b) The client's physical/sociocultural environment
   c) Clinical signs and symptoms, treatment for diagnosis
3. How will you find the answers to your questions? What is your plan for finding the needed information?

Now, compare your answers with the rest of your group. Through this discussion with the group, you will be sharing knowledge and learning from each other. Consolidate the group's work on the Tutorial Session Sheet. The Tutorial Session Sheet keeps track of the group's learning issues and the group's plan for finding answers. As you go along with the different parts of the case study, you will be answering questions and learning issues, as well as generating more questions and learning issues. You can update the Tutorial Session Sheet as you go along by "crossing out" the learning issues when answers have been found and adding new learning issues as they arise. An abbreviated Tutorial Session Sheet example is provided (Figure 3-1b).

The knowledge you have already gives you some idea of how you will address this case. For example, medical management of a right Colles fracture, a type of wrist fracture, requires immobilization for a period of time. Pain and swelling may be present. Secondary complications of prolonged immobilization include decreased strength and decreased ROM in the fore-arm, wrist, and hand. This would limit a person's ability to use the upper extremity for functional tasks, limiting independence in activities of daily living (ADL) and instrumental activities of daily living (IADL), and interfering with role performance and valued occupations.

This should get you to start thinking about the types of assessments that you need to perform to establish a

TUTORIAL SESSION SHEET

Case Study (Pt. Name, Dx.): Maggie; Right Colles Fracture, 2 days post

Group Members' Names: _____

Facts/Knowledge

What do you already know that will help you to approach this case?

1. Individual client–roles, tasks, activities
2. The client's physical/sociocultural environment
3. Clinical signs and symptoms, treatment for diagnosis

Learning Issues

What questions do you need to ask to learn about:

1. Individual client–roles, tasks, activities
2. The client's physical/sociocultural environment
3. Clinical signs and symptoms, treatment for diagnosis

Actions/Steps to Learn

What are the plans to find the answers to your questions?

Figure 3–1a. Tutorial session sheet.

Tutorial Session Sheet Example

Case Study (Pt. Name, Dx.): Maggie; Right Colles Fracture, 2 days post

Facts/Knowledge	Learning Issues	Actions/Steps to Learn
What do you already know that will help you to approach this case?	What questions do you need to ask to learn about:	What are the plans to find the answers to your questions?
1. Individual client - roles, tasks, activities	1. Individual client - roles, tasks, activities	
2. The client's physical/sociocultural environment	2. The client's physical/sociocultural environment	
3. Clinical signs and symptoms, treatment for diagnosis	3. Clinical signs and symptoms, treatment for diagnosis	
Part 1	**Part 1**	**Part 1**
61-year-old female - shops	~~What are Maggie's roles? Prior level of Function? Living situation? Hand dominance?~~	Interview Maggie
Right Colles fracture - type of wrist fracture	How did she fall?	Review medical record
Fractures immobilized	~~Medical History~~	Consult with physician
Fractures cause pain, edema	Precautions	Consult orthopedic textbooks and OT textbooks
Fractures limit ability to use upper extremity functionally	Medical management post fractures	Consult with local occupational therapist
	Possible complications	Consult other instructors
Part 2	Prognosis to return to prior level of function	**Part 2**
Lives alone	~~Occupational Therapy Evaluation and Treatment Concerns~~	Additional Plans:
Was independent in ADL and IADL, caring for dog and cat also	**Part 2**	Perform occupational therapy assessments
Works for her son	Additional Learning Issues:	**Part 3**
Active in church, Craft Bazaar and Fish Dinner	Tasks and activities that Maggie needs to do to resume roles	
Anxious about present situation	**Part 3**	
Immobilized in plaster cast		
Physician restricted activities		
Part 3		

Figure 3-1b. Tutorial session sheet example.

treatment plan. As you read Part 2 of this case, continue to think about the occupational therapy areas of concern and appropriate assessments.

CHOOSING ASSESSMENTS

Part 2

On your first visit to see Maggie, you interview her and find out the following information. Maggie was in excellent health prior to this injury. Maggie's son, Fred, lives in the next town. She works part-time in her son's accounting office. A widow, she lives alone with her cat and her dog. Maggie is concerned that since she lives alone she needs to be able to do all the cooking, cleaning, and care for her dog and cat. Her son is only able to come to her home every other day or every 3 days to assist with some of these activities.

Maggie is concerned about her present situation. She is right-handed and states that although she tries her best, she is not able to do very much for herself. Maggie has been very active in her local church organization. Maggie always heads up the Christmas crafts bazaar. Part of her responsibilities for the bazaar include organizing and teaching at craft nights. Maggie also has been one of the primary cooks for the annual fish dinner held just before Easter. She states that the church especially needs her this year as the other primary cook is moving to another state. She also doesn't want to let the church organization down.

In the emergency room on October 27, the emergency room physician performed a closed reduction and applied a plaster cast from mid humeral level to the metacarpophalangeal (MP) joints of the right hand. The elbow is casted in approximately 90 degrees of elbow flexion and the wrist is casted in approximately 30 degrees of wrist flexion. Maggie states that the physician has instructed her to stay home for the next 2 weeks and not to drive or do any housework. This is confirmed when you speak to the physician.

Analysis of Part 2

This initial interview with Maggie gives you more information for developing the evaluation and treatment plan.

- You find out some of Maggie's roles—mother, worker, volunteer, pet owner. (narrative reasoning)
- The interview reveals Maggie's health status and prior level of function—excellent health and independent as she lived alone. (narrative reasoning)
- In view of the prognosis for recovery post-fracture and the prior level of independence, the dis-

charge plan would be to return the client to her identified roles and prior level of function. (conditional reasoning)

- You also learn about her present functional status—she is unable to use her dominant upper extremity as it is immobilized in a cast. This limits her ability in ADL and IADL. Further, the physician has restricted her activity. (procedural reasoning)
- Maggie is concerned about her activity limitations but is motivated to do things for herself. (interactional reasoning)
- You find out about some of her support systems—her son can assist every other day or every 3 days. (pragmatic reasoning)

Now to continue to find out more about Maggie, develop a plan for further evaluation by answering the following questions. When choosing assessments, keep in mind the time constraints you may have when in an actual clinic.

Questions: Part 2

1. What are the occupational therapy concerns? (What performance areas and performance components are of concern?)
2. What specific assessments would you use (Formal assessments, informal assessments, observations, interview)?
3. How will you use the assessment results?

Compare and discuss your answers with your group. Consolidate the group's work and enter on the Case Study Evaluation Plan worksheet. This worksheet can be copied and shared with your other classmates so they can learn from your group (Figure 3-2a).

Now that you have established a plan for evaluating Maggie, Part 3 gives you the evaluation results. As this is a "paper case," all of your specific questions about the individual client may not be answered, limiting your ability to develop an appropriate treatment plan. In a "real case" you would find the answers to these questions by asking the client, significant other, physician, nurse, social worker, or other professional. Therefore, with these "paper cases" you may find the answers to your questions by:

1. Addressing additional questions to the physician, nurse, social worker, or other professional. In these "paper cases" these roles will be played by your instructor or other designated person.
2. Addressing additional questions to the person in your group (or other designee) chosen to be the client. In this particular case the chosen person will play Maggie, a 61-year-old woman with a right Colles fracture. Maggie can tell you more

CASE STUDY EVALUATION PLAN

Case Study (Pt. Name, Dx.):   *Maggie; Right Colles Fracture, 2 days post*

Group Members' Names: _____

Concerns/Performance Components/Areas	Assessments	How will assessment results be used?

Figure 3-2a. Case study evaluation plan.

CASE STUDY EVALUATION PLAN

Case Study (Pt. Name, Dx.): Maggie; Right Colles Fracture, 2 days post

Group Members' Names: _____

Concerns/Performance Components/Areas	Assessments	How will assessment results be used?
1. Maggie's perception of her strengths and weaknesses and her priorities for therapy.	1. Canadian Occupational Therapy Performance Measure (COPM) or other informal interview tool.	1. Set client-centered goals for therapy; establish rapport; gain better understanding of Maggie's occupational context.
2. Decreased ADL performance due to right (dominant) upper extremity (UE) in cast.	2. Observe Maggie attempting to perform ADL tasks; Klein-Bell ADL assessment; self-report; Functional Independence Measure (FIM).	2. Assess potential for teaching compensatory techniques or use of adaptive equipment; determine components of ADL tasks causing difficulty; determine baseline for therapy.
3. Unable to carry out worker/volunteer roles.	3. Interview Maggie to determine specific worker/volunteer tasks and activities.	3. Determine readiness to return to work and volunteer duties; assess potential for adapting tasks and activities.
4. Unable to participate in leisure interests.	4. Interest checklist; formal or informal interview.	4. Determine realistic leisure interests; Assess potential for adapting leisure activities.
5. Sensorimotor concerns (motor): potential for edema, stiffness, and Reflex Sympathetic Dystrophy (RSD) in right hand; Potential for frozen right shoulder.	5. Active/passive range of motion (A/PROM) assessment of proximal interphalangeal (PIP) and distal interphalangeal (DIP) joints of right hand; circumferential edema measurements of digits; pain assessment (1 to 10 scale); A/PROM measurements of right shoulder.	5. Set baseline for therapy; develop treatment plan which includes management of edema and home exercise program (HEP) to maintain range of motion (ROM) and prevent complications.
6. Sensorimotor concerns (sensory): possible sensory loss or altered sensation due to pressure on nerves from swelling or tight cast.	6. Sensory evaluation to exposed areas; observe cast for fit, look for areas of redness where cast is pressing against skin.	6. Set baseline for therapy; make suggestions for alterations of cast if necessary; determine need to teach compensatory techniques or sensory reeducation program if sensation is impaired or absent.
7. Psychosocial and cognitive concerns: potential for depression due to loss of role performance and feelings of helplessness.	7. Formal or informal interview; observe Maggie during evaluation session; speak with family members and other rehab team members (social worker, psychologist).	7. Determine Maggie's motivation for therapy; assess ability to follow directions and carry out HEP; set realistic goals appropriate for Maggie's cognitive and emotional status.

Figure 3-2b. Case study evaluation plan example.

about her meaningful occupations or her roles, tasks, activities, interests, and priorities (these can be pretend) to assist you in developing your treatment plan and selecting appropriate therapeutic activities.

Now move on to Part 3 to find out the evaluation results.

DEVELOPING A TREATMENT PLAN

Part 3

You evaluated Maggie and found the following:

Maggie is cognitively intact and motivated to be independent. Maggie is proud as she describes her success at figuring out how to open the foil packet of cat food with her left hand so that she could feed her cat. She is unable to don some types of blouses and dresses over the cast and is not able to don pants or skirts with closures. She requires minimal assistance to don a house dress, underpants and socks. She is unable to don her bra, panty hose, or tie her shoes/sneakers. Because of the inability to use her dominant right hand, Maggie is unable to manage buttons, has difficulty feeding herself with her nondominant left hand (spills food on herself frequently), requires minimal assist with personal hygiene after toileting, sponge bathing, and brushing her teeth. She requires maximal assistance in simple meal preparation. Maggie states she is able to get herself some simple food items, such as prepared foods (prepared by her son's wife) from plastic containers. She is dependent in household chores such as cleaning.

Through further interview, you learn that much of Maggie's work at her son's office involves working with Excel, a spreadsheet program. She has a computer at home and is an avid Internet user. She tells you that it is difficult to use the computer now because she cannot use her right hand.

Tasks associated with her responsibilities as chairperson of the Christmas craft bazaar include phoning church members to inform them of meeting times, craft supplies they will be required to bring, and delegation of other responsibilities such as making refreshments, teaching certain crafts, and clean-up duties. She is having difficulty using her old style rotary dial telephone to keep in touch with the other church volunteers.

Maggie complains of (c/o) moderate pain in her right upper extremity, mainly the wrist and fingers. She rates her pain an 8 on a scale of 1 to 10. She describes it as a burning, throbbing type of pain. Severe edema is noted in all of the digits of the right hand (approximately two times the size of the left hand). She has a great deal of difficulty flexing her fingers to make a fist (the cast restricts the MP motion). She is unable to oppose her thumb to her index or any other finger. She is unable to hold any objects in her right hand because of the cast. She states that at times her hand feels numb and other times she has paresthesia. The fingers are discolored, a dusky reddish color.

In your conversation with the home health coordinator and the social worker, you find out that Maggie's insurance will cover home health occupational therapy for up to 3 months for the purpose of improving independence in ADLs.

In order to use a client-centered approach, select one person in your group to be Maggie. This person can then tell you more about her roles, tasks, activities, interests, and priorities (this can be pretend) to assist you in developing your treatment plan and selecting appropriate therapeutic activities.

Analysis of Part 3

Once you have completed the evaluation process, use this information to develop a treatment plan. When developing a treatment plan, keep in mind factors that will affect the implementation of the treatment plan or the selection of treatment methods and specific activities and modalities. These may include:

1. Immediate concerns that may require immediate action and/or consultation with another health care practitioner.

2. Precautions and safety concerns.

3. Deficits that affect participation in therapy which may not be deficits specifically addressed in the occupational therapy plan of treatment, but will influence how the plan is implemented. For example, if Maggie had severely impaired short-term memory, you would not provide therapy to improve her memory. However, if you wanted to implement a home activity program, Maggie would not have the potential to learn this program. Your efforts should focus on educating a cognitively aware significant other to help Maggie carry out the home activity program.

To summarize, the interviews and assessments provided you with the following information to enable you to develop a comprehensive treatment plan:

1. The clinical signs and symptoms of severe edema in the right digits, discoloration of the right digits, and sensory deficits of intermittent numbness and paresthesia indicate a problem that needs immediate attention. These problems suggest the cast is fitting too tightly, compromising neurovascular integrity. This probably was caused by an increase in swelling after the cast was applied. The

physician needs to be contacted immediately for cast removal and replacement, otherwise permanent damage may result (procedural reasoning; pragmatic reasoning).

2. You found out specific information on Maggie's functional status, strengths, and limitations (procedural reasoning). You also found out about Maggie's priorities (narrative reasoning) and motivation to be independent (interactional reasoning).

3. You found out about one of the physical resources that Maggie has that may help her return to one of her roles—a home computer (pragmatic reasoning).

4. You found out that Maggie's insurance will cover home health occupational therapy for up to 3 months. You realize that occupational therapy may not be needed continuously for this period of time. Maggie is motivated to be independent and learns quickly. She will learn one-handed techniques, become independent using compensatory techniques, perform a home activity program very quickly, and can be put on hold status until the cast is removed (pragmatic reasoning).

With this information, you can develop a treatment plan. For learning purposes, you will be required to complete an expanded treatment plan format. This expanded format will require identification of the following:

Deficits

Deficits should be written as functional problem statements. The functional problem statement should focus on a performance area (i.e., self-care, work, or leisure). The statement should identify the level of assistance the client needs to complete or participate in the performance area. A statement about a limitation in a performance component may be used to clarify why the client requires assistance in the performance area.

Example: The client requires moderate assist (assistance level) with upper body dressing (performance area) due to poor strength in the left upper extremity (performance component).

Stage-Specific Cause

This is an identification of the cause or reason for the deficit at this specific time or stage post injury or illness.

It is important to identify the stage-specific cause of a deficit to assist with choosing specific frame(s) of reference and treatment method(s). To illustrate this, consider this example.

A client who suffered a left humeral fracture was referred to you approximately 5 weeks post injury. The physician has ordered OT to evaluate and treat and has given the okay to start active range of motion (AROM) activities. You assess AROM in the client's left shoulder and find that AROM in shoulder flexion is limited to 0 to 70 degrees, while shoulder abduction is limited to 0 to 60 degrees. The client complains of pain in the shoulder and inability to use the left arm for functional tasks.

You identify a deficit as "AROM in left shoulder flexion 0 to 70 degrees and abduction of 0 to 60 degrees limiting functional use of left upper extremity." The stage-specific cause is pain and decreased muscle strength. At this stage, the prognosis is good to increase AROM in the left shoulder thereby improving functional use. You decide to use a biomechanical frame of reference providing activities to increase AROM.

Now, consider if you saw this same client 1 year post injury and found the AROM and passive range of motion (PROM) limitations in left shoulder flexion of 0 to 90 degrees and abduction 0 to 80 degrees with a hard end feel at end of ROM. The prognosis for improving the ROM is extremely limited, as the stage-specific cause of the ROM limitation would be soft tissue contractures. The client still has difficulty with activities requiring reaching with the left upper extremity (LUE) such as reaching to get dishes from an overhead cupboard. At this point, because of the stage-specific cause, you know you will not be able to make considerable improvement in ROM so you decide to use a rehabilitation frame of reference, providing adaptive equipment or teaching compensatory methods.

Short-Term Goals

Short-term goals (STGs) can be achieved in a relatively short period of time and are the building blocks to achieving long-term goals (LTGs).

Borcherding (2000) outlines the FEAST Method for goal writing. This method can be used to write both STGs and LTGs.

The components of the FEAST Method are:

- F is for *function*: identifies the performance area that the goal relates to.

- E is for *expectation*: this sets the expectation of who will accomplish what. The expectation is usually for the client but in some cases may be for a significant other in his or her role of assisting or caring for the client.

- A is for *action*: this identifies the specific action the client (or in some cases the significant other) will do.

- S is for *specific condition*: this identifies the specific conditions in which the client will perform the action (e.g., at wheelchair level, or using a reacher).

- T is for *timeline*: this identifies a time frame for achieving a goal. In physical disabilities settings, the time frame is not always a part of the goal statement, however the time frame is stated in the treatment plan (e.g., STGs to be accomplished in 2 weeks).

Functional Outcomes or Long-Term Goals

The functional outcome, or LTGs addresses a performance area. LTG's are established for the time frame the client is expected to be treated in a particular setting. The FEAST method of writing goals also applies to LTGs.

Treatment Methods

Treatment methods are the OT tools and/or modalities used in treatment. Examples of treatment methods include strengthening activities, education in energy conservation techniques, and environmental modifications.

Rationale

Rationale explains why treatment methods work. It is important to understand the rationale behind a treatment method because you often will have to explain how a treatment works to clients, significant others, physicians, and third-party payers.

Treatment Approach(es)/Frame(s) of Reference

Treatment approaches and frames of reference provide a way of looking at a situation or problem and provide suggestions for specific treatment. Common frames of reference used in physical disability treatment include the biomechanical, rehabilitative, and neurodevelopmental including the Rood, Brunnstrom, Bobath, and Proprioceptive Neuromuscular Facilitation (PNF) approaches. Often these approaches are used in conjunction with OT models such as the Model of Human Occupation and the Canadian Occupational Performance Model to provide more of an individualized, client-centered approach.

Specific Activity/Modality

In this section you must be very specific in describing the activity and how you will present the activity. Describe how the client will be positioned, how the activity will be positioned, who will be educated in a home activity program, how long the client will participate in the activity, as well as any other information pertinent to presentation of the activity. Activity analysis skills and ability to adapt activities and/or the environment are instrumental for this section.

The treatment plans that you write in the clinic will not contain all the information that is included on this treatment plan. Generally, treatment plans in physical disabilities will include: deficits, STGs, LTGs, and treatment methods. This expanded treatment plan format is for learning purposes.

Questions: Part 3

Answer the following questions, then discuss your answers with your group.

1. What are the deficit areas that the OT treatment plan will address? State deficits in measurable terms.

2. What are the stage-specific causes of these deficits (what is the reason for each of these deficits)?

3. What are the OT STGs? State in measurable terms.

4. What are the projected functional outcomes (LTGs)?

5. What treatment methods will be used to achieve the goal and what is the rationale for this method (why will the method work)?

6. What is the frame of reference for each treatment method or approach?

7. What specific activity(ies) will you as the therapist use and how can this (these) activity(ies) be graded? In this section you must be very specific in describing how you will present the activity. Describe how the client will be positioned; how the activity will be positioned, who will be educated in a home activity program, how long the client will participate in the activity, etc.

For subsequent case studies, your group will consolidate your answers and enter the information on the Case Study Treatment Plan Sheet to develop a treatment plan. For this case study, look at the example provided (Figures 3-3a and 3-3b). Were your answers to the questions similar in nature to the Case Study Treatment Plan Example? You may use this example as a guide for subsequent case studies. In some of the case studies you will be requested to complete a tutorial session sheet, a case study evaluation plan sheet, and a treatment plan sheet. For some of the case studies you will be requested to complete one or more of the above listed worksheets and/or answer specific questions related to the case and treatment planning for that case.

Keep in mind that there is not an absolute "gold standard" when developing the case study evaluation plans and/or the treatment plans. Choice of assessments, wording of goal statements, choice of treatment methods, and selection and grading of specific activities may vary. Realize however, that there is always room for improvement through collaboration and constructive comments which will help to refine your treatment planning skills.

CASE STUDY TREATMENT PLAN EXAMPLE

Page 1

Case Study (Client Name; Dx.): Maggie; Right Colles Fracture, 2 days post

Deficits	Stage-Specific Cause	Short-Term Goals	Relates to which deficit	Functional Outcomes	Relates to which STG
1. Spills food when eating with left hand.	1. Unable to use dominant right hand. Presently using non-dominant left hand.	1. Client will use adapted utensil to feed self with non-dominant left hand without spilling.	See # preceding short-term goal	1. Independent feeding with right hand.	See # preceding functional outcome
2. Minimal assist with personal hygiene (toilet hygiene, brushing teeth).	2. Dominant right UE is non-functional secondary to immobilization and pain.	2. Independent with personal hygiene (toileting, brushing teeth) using one-hand techniques and adaptive aids.		2. Independent with personal hygiene.	
3. Minimal assist with sponge bathing.	3. Same	3. Independent sponge bathing using one-hand techniques and adaptive aids.		3. Independent bathing.	
4. Minimal assist with donning/doffing house dress, underpants, socks.	4. Same	4. Independent donning/doffing house dress, underpants, socks using compensatory techniques.		4. *and* 5. Independent dressing.	
5. Dependent in donning bra, panty hose, shoes/sneakers.	5. Same	5. Minimal assist donning/doffing bra, panty hose, sneakers using adaptive aides/compensatory techniques.		6. Independent in simple meal preparation.	
6. Maximal assist with meal preparation.	6. Same	6. Minimal assist simple meal preparation using adaptive aides/compensatory techniques.		7. Independent in performing chairperson role—organizing and managing all chairperson tasks for Craft Bazaar using adaptive aides/compensatory techniques.	
7. Unable to perform volunteer role of chairperson of Craft Bazaar.	7. Same	7. Independent in using phone to contact volunteers to organize Craft Bazaar using adaptive aides/compensatory techniques.			

Figure 3-3a. Case study treatment plan example—Page 1.

CASE STUDY TREATMENT PLAN EXAMPLE

Case Study (Client Name; Dx.): Maggie; Right Colles Fracture, 2 days post

Page 1 continued

Deficits	Stage-Specific Cause	Short-Term Goals	Relates to which deficit	Functional Outcomes	Relates to which STG
8. Unable to perform worker role/tasks; using computer to manage accounting files.	8. Same; unable to travel to workplace.	8. Independent in using home computer to perform work tasks using adaptive aids and compensatory techniques.	See # preceding short-term goal	8. Independent in work activities at workplace using adaptive aids and compensatory techniques.	See # preceding functional outcome
9. Potential for muscle wasting in right wrist extensors and flexors limiting functional use of right UE.	9. Immobilization in cast.	9. Client will perform home exercise program (HEP) of isometric exercises independently.		9. *and* 10. Client will use RUE functionally for light daily living tasks.	
10. Potential for active range of motion and muscle strength to decrease in right shoulder which will limit functional use of right UE.	10. Inability to use right UE for functional activities.	10. Client will perform home activity program independently, to prevent decrease in AROM and muscle strength in right shoulder motions and muscle groups.		11. Eliminate edema in right hand to enable functional use of right UE.	
11. Client has severe edema in digits in right digits with potential for contractures which will limit functional use of right UE.	11. Immobilization in cast.	11. Client will independently perform self retrograde massage.			
		STGs To be accomplished in approximately 2 weeks.		LTGs To be accomplished in approximately 2 months.	

Figure 3-3a. Case study treatment plan example—Page 1 continued.

CASE STUDY TREATMENT PLAN EXAMPLE

Case Study (Client Name; Dx.): Maggie; Right Colles Fracture, 2 days post

Short-Term Goals	Methods	Rationale	Tx Approach/ Frame of Reference	Specific Activity/ Modality
1. Client will use adapted utensil to feed self with nondominant left hand without spilling.	1. Provide textured built up handle to compensate for decreased manipulation of nondominant hand. Provided adaptive aids and educate in the use of compensatory techniques for cutting, scooping, and spearing foods with one hand.	1. Textured handle will enable better manipulation of utensil. Compensate for lost function of RUE.	Rehabilitative Approach (Use of compensatory technique and adaptive aids.)	1. Client will be provided with textured handle for utensils (plastazote). Client will be instructed how to hold utensils. Client will practice using adapted spoon with left hand to spoon water from bowl to glass. Client will be provided with rocker knife and dycem and educated in use. Client will practice cutting food using these adaptive aids.
2. Independent personal hygiene (toileting, brushing teeth) using one-hand techniques and adaptive aids.	2., 3., 4., 5., and 6. Educate client in use of compensatory technique and adaptive aids which compensate for lost function of RUE.	2., 3., 4., 5., and 6. Compensate for lost function of RUE.		2. Client will be educated in and practice one-hand technique of opening toothpaste and applying toothpaste to brush.
3. Independent sponge bathing using one-hand techniques and adaptive aids.				3. Client will be provided with "octopus" suction cup to hold soap and educated in how to soap wash cloth using left hand only. Client will be educated in wringing wash cloth with one hand (pressing it against side of sink). Client will practice these techniques with assist and verbal cues from therapist.
4. Independent donning/doffing house dress, underpants, socks using compensatory techniques.				4. Client will be educated in and helped to select type of clothing that will fit easily over cast. Client will be educated in one hand techniques for donning/doffing housedress, underpants, and socks. Client will practice these techniques with assistance and verbal cues from therapist.

Figure 3-3b. Case study treatment plan example—Page 2.

CASE STUDY TREATMENT PLAN EXAMPLE

Page 2 continued

Case Study (Client Name; Dx.): Maggie; Right Colles Fracture, 2 days post

Short-Term Goals	Methods	Rationale	Tx Approach/ Frame of Reference	Specific Activity/ Modality
5. Minimal assist donning/doffing bra, panty hose, shoes, sneakers using adaptive aides/ compensatory techniques. 6. Minimal assistance in simple meal preparation using adaptive aides/compensatory techniques. 7. Independent in using phone to contact volunteers to organize Craft Bazaar using adaptive aides/compensatory techniques. 8. Independent in using home computer to perform work tasks using adaptive aids and compensatory techniques.	7. Educate client in use of compensatory technique and adaptive aids *which compensate for lost function of right UE.* 8. Educate client in use of compensatory technique and adaptive aids *which compensate for lost function of right UE and restricted ability to travel to work.*	7. Compensate for lost function of right UE. 8. Compensate for lost function of right UE and restricted ability to travel to work.	Rehabilitation Approach	5. Client will be provided elastic laces for shoes and sneakers. Client will be educated in donning/doffing of shoes/sneakers and will practice with assistance and verbal cues from therapist. Client will be educate in one hand technique (hooking bra in front) for donning/doffing bra and will practice technique with therapist assistance and cues. 6. Client will be educated in use of pre-packaged food, compensatory techniques to open packages. Client's cutting board will be adapted with stainless steel nails and jig for stabilizing foods when cutting or spreading butter, etc. Client will be educated to use lightweight, small pots, pans for cooking. Client will practice simple meal preparation with assistance and verbal cues from therapist. 7. Client will be assisted to obtain speaker phone with large buttons for "dialing." Phone will be positioned in an easily accessible place for client, in an area where other volunteer work supplies can be

Figure 3-3b. Case study treatment plan example—Page 2 continued.

CASE STUDY TREATMENT PLAN EXAMPLE

Case Study (Client Name; Dx.): Maggie; Right Colles Fracture, 2 days post

Page 2 continued

Short-Term Goals	Methods	Rationale	Tx Approach/ Frame of Reference	Specific Activity/ Modality
9. Client will perform home exercise program (HEP) of isometric exercises with minimal verbal cues. 10. Client will perform home activity program with minimal assist, to prevent decrease in AROM and muscle strength in right shoulder motions and muscle groups. 11. Client will independently perform self retrograde massage.	9. Educate client in isometric exercise for right wrist musculature. 10. Client will be educated in activities/exercises to move UE through all of shoulder motions. 11. Applying pressure distally to proximally through massage to the hand.	9. Active contraction of muscle fibers will maintain muscle bulk. 10. Stretch of muscles and connective tissue through full range of motion daily prevents shortening of these tissues. Stress (weight) provided by weight of cast will maintain or increase muscle bulk. 11. Will prevent filtration of fluids from capillaries into the interstitial tissues and assists with blood and lymph flow.	Biomechanical Approach	placed (e.g., phone numbers, checklists, etc.). Client will be educated in using the phone with one hand techniques. Client will be assisted to list chairperson tasks and delegate duties to various volunteers (e.g., purchasing of supplies, teaching crafts, etc.). 8. The client's home computer will be adapted for left hand use (e.g., mouse function will be changed to use for left hand; if appropriate, computer tower will be repositioned on the left side for ease in turning on/off and inserting disks). Client will be educated in sending and receiving work files via email. 9. Client will be educated in technique of performing isometric exercises for right wrist musculature. Client will perform ten repetitions of isometric exercises three times per day. 10. Therapist will provide written and video taped guide to home activity program of exercises to move UE through all of shoulder motions. Client will be instructed in how to perform home activity program.
STGs To be accomplished in approximately 2 weeks.				

Figure 3-3b. Case study treatment plan example—Page 2 continued.

CASE STUDY TREATMENT PLAN EXAMPLE

Page 2 continued

Case Study (Client Name; Dx.): Maggie; Right Colles Fracture, 2 days post

Short-Term Goals	Methods	Rationale	Tx Approach/ Frame of Reference	Specific Activity/ Modality
				(Ten repetitions of each exercise, three times per day). 11. Therapist will perform retrograde massage to the hand each treatment session. Client will be educated in self retrograde massage and instructed to perform three times per day.

Figure 3-3b. Case study treatment plan example—Page 2 continued.

Chapter 4

Maggie

Accountant's Assistant with a Right Colles Fracture, 6 Weeks Postoperative

---

PART 1

Maggie is a 61-year-old female referred to outpatient occupational therapy on December 9th, with a diagnosis of right Colles fracture. Maggie fell while shopping at her neighborhood department store on October 27th. The physician has ordered gentle AROM for the right hand and wrist and ADL training.

Determine learning issues and plan using Tutorial Session Sheet.

TUTORIAL SESSION SHEET

Case Study (Pt. Name, Dx.): Maggie; Right Colles Fracture, 6 weeks post

Group Members' Names: _____

Facts/Knowledge

What do you already know that will help you to approach this case?

1. Individual client—roles, tasks, activities
2. The client's physical/sociocultural environment
3. Clinical signs and symptoms, treatment for diagnosis

Learning Issues

What questions do you need to ask to learn about:

1. Individual client—roles, tasks, activities
2. The client's physical/sociocultural environment
3. Clinical signs and symptoms, treatment for diagnosis

Actions/Steps to Learn

What are the plans to find the answers to your questions?

PART 2

On your first visit to see Maggie, you interview her and find out the following information. Maggie has been in excellent health prior to this injury. Maggie's son, Fred, lives in the next town. She works part-time in her son's accounting office. A widow, she lives alone with her cat and her dog. Maggie is concerned that since she lives alone she needs to be able to do all the cooking, cleaning, and care for her dog and cat. Her son is only able to come to her home every other day or every 3 days to assist with some of these activities.

She is anxious to get back to her son's office to work. She says she will need to be able to use her right hand to write, type, answer phones, and lift office supplies of up to 10 pounds. Maggie has been very active in her local church organization. Maggie always heads up the Christmas crafts bazaar. Part of her responsibilities for the bazaar include organizing and teaching at craft nights. She is also anxious to get working on the Christmas craft bazaar, which will be held next week. She has been helping by teaching some of the other ladies how to make certain crafts, however, she wants to contribute her own creations. Maggie also has been one of the primary cooks for the annual fish dinner held just before Easter. She states that the church especially needs her this year because the other primary cook is moving to another state and that she doesn't want to let the church organization down.

In the emergency room on October 27th, the emergency room physician performed a closed reduction and applied a plaster cast from mid humeral level to the MP joints of the right hand. The elbow was casted in approximately 90 degrees of elbow flexion and the wrist was casted in approximately 30 degrees of wrist flexion. That cast was removed on November 17th and replaced with a shorter cast from just distal to the elbow to the metacarpalphalangeal (MCP) joints. This cast was removed on December 8th.

Determine evaluation plan using the Case Study Evaluation Plan worksheet.

CASE STUDY EVALUATION PLAN SHEET

Case Study (Pt. Name, Dx.): *Maggie; Right Colles Fracture, 6 weeks post*

Group Members' Names: _____

Concerns/Performance Components/Areas	Assessments	How will assessment results be used?

PART 3

You have evaluated Maggie and have found the following:

Maggie is cognitively intact and motivated to be independent. Maggie is proud as she describes her success at "figuring out" how to open the foil packet of cat food with her left hand so that she can feed her cat. She states that since she lives alone she needs to be able to do all the cooking, cleaning, and care for her dog and cat efficiently. At the present time, her son has been helping her to do many of these activities because she was only able to use her left hand.

Maggie has been wearing large, loose-fitting pullover blouses, loose-fitting elastic waistband pants, and sneakers with velcro closures which she has donned and doffed herself. She prefers to wear tighter-fitting clothes, and most of her clothes have closures (buttons, zippers, snaps, and shoelaces). She wants to be able to dress up in nice outfits to be able to go to work and attend church functions.

While she had her cast on, she was feeding herself with her nondominant left hand. She continues to do this for the most part because when using her right hand, the hand "pains her and gets tired quickly." For the same reason she has been brushing her teeth, combing her hair, and doing most of her self-care and light daily living tasks with her left hand.

She is able to prepare simple meals for herself (e.g., cold cereal, simple sandwiches, prepared foods [prepared by her son's wife] from plastic containers, and microwave dinners). She states her son "opens" food containers for her, leaving them loosely shut. She does light cleaning but her daughter-in-law has been helping with more thorough, heavier cleaning tasks.

Through further interview, you learn that Maggie has been working from home. She has a computer at home and learned how to adapt the computer mouse for left hand use to manage the Excel files, a spreadsheet program. She is able to email files back and forth. She is anxious to return to work, as she misses her work colleagues.

Maggie tells you she has been able to use her large button speaker phone to contact church volunteers and delegate some of her duties. She tells you some of the tasks she is responsible for as primary cook of the annual fish dinner include ordering food, preparing food, and directing other volunteers to prepare food. She is concerned about her ability to manage large pots and pans, large containers of food, and to cut raw fish and vegetables. She does not have to serve food or clean up.

Maggie c/o moderate pain in her RUE, mainly the wrist and fingers. She rates her pain as a five on a scale of 1 to 10. Minimal to moderate edema is noted in all of the digits of the right hand and wrist. AROM in Maggie's right wrist measures 0 to 10 degrees in wrist extension, 0 to 30 degrees in wrist flexion, 0 to 5 degrees of radial and ulnar deviation, full pronation, but supination is limited to 0 to 50 degrees. She is able to make a full fist however, she has not been able to hold any object heavier than a hair brush. She was able to grasp a pen and write her name but legibility was poor.

What will you do to help Maggie?

In order to use a client-centered approach, select one person in your group to "be" Maggie. This person can then tell you more about her roles, tasks, activities, interests, and priorities (this can be pretend) to assist you in developing your treatment plan and selecting appropriate therapeutic activities.

Develop a treatment plan using the Case Study Treatment Plan sheets.

Case Study Treatment Plan Sheet

Page 1

Case Study (Client Name; Dx.): *Maggie; Right Colles Fracture, 6 weeks post*

Group Members' Names: _____

Deficits	Stage-Specific Cause	Short-Term Goals	Relates to which deficit	Functional Outcomes	Relates to which STG

CASE STUDY TREATMENT PLAN SHEET

Page 2

Case Study (Client Name; Dx.): Maggie; Right Colles Fracture, 6 weeks post

Group Members' Names: _____

Short-Term Goals	Methods	Rationale	Tx Approach/ Frame of Reference	Specific Activity/ Modality

Chapter

5

Ida

Teacher with a Right Humeral Fracture, 6 Days Postoperative

PART 1

Ida is a 55-year-old female referred to home health OT on October 20th with status post (s/p) right humeral fracture. Ida is an elementary school teacher. She fell at school on October 14th. She lives with her husband who is retired. The physician has ordered OT evaluation and treatment.

TUTORIAL SESSION SHEET

Case Study (Pt. Name, Dx.): Ida; Right Humeral Fracture, 6 days post

Group Members' Names: _____

Facts/Knowledge	Learning Issues	Actions/Steps to Learn
What do you already know that will help you to approach this case?	What questions do you need to ask to learn about:	What are the plans to find the answers to your questions?
1. Individual client—roles, tasks, activities	1. Individual client—roles, tasks, activities	
2. The client's physical/sociocultural environment	2. The client's physical/sociocultural environment	
3. Clinical signs and symptoms, treatment for diagnosis	3. Clinical signs and symptoms, treatment for diagnosis	

PART 2

Ida has been in excellent health. She has had no significant health problems. Ida fractured her humerus at the mid-humeral level. There was no surgical procedure. The physician has immobilized her RUE in a sling and swathe. The physician is allowing her to remove the sling and swathe for bathing only and cautioned her not to move the arm in any way. The physician has advised Ida to stay home from work for 2 weeks and not to do any chores at home.

You call the physician for specific orders, which are Codman's pendulum exercises and isometric exercises for the right shoulder as well as ADL training.

CASE STUDY EVALUATION PLAN

Case Study (Pt. Name, Dx.): *Ida; Right Humeral Fracture, 6 days post*

Group Members' Names: _____

Concerns/Performance Components/Areas	Assessments	How will assessment results be used?

PART 3

Ida requires moderate to maximal assistance with bathing and dressing, and minimal assistance with toileting activities, managing clothing and cleaning herself. She is unable to manage any clothes fasteners. Ida states she is right handed and is responsible for all the cooking, cleaning, and laundering in her home. She is unable to perform these activities at the present time. Ida is very concerned about how she will care for herself, how she will manage her household activities, and also about how she will be able to manage when she returns to work.

Ida complains of moderate pain in her right upper arm. She rates the pain level as an 8 on a scale of 1 to 10. She states this pain increases when she gets in and out of bed, up and down from the toilet, and in and out of the car. She also complains of increased pain when the sling and swathe are removed for bathing especially when she tries to straighten her elbow.

Ida has moderate edema in the right hand which restricts her ability to make a tight fist. Her RUE is ecchymotic on the lateral aspect of the upper arm. AROM in right wrist motions is within functional limits (WFL). AROM in the right elbow is 75 degrees to 115 degrees. Sensation for light touch is intact throughout the RUE. The strength and AROM in Ida's left arm is within normal limits (WNL). What will you do to help Ida?

In order to use a client-centered approach, select one person in your group to "be" Ida. This person can then tell you more about her roles, tasks, activities, interests, and priorities (this can be pretend) to assist you in developing your treatment plan and selecting appropriate therapeutic activities.

CASE STUDY TREATMENT PLAN SHEET

Page 1

Case Study (Client Name; Dx.): Ida; Right Humeral Fracture, 6 days post

Group Members' Names: _____

Deficits	Stage-Specific Cause	Short-Term Goals	Relates to which deficit	Functional Outcomes	Relates to which STG

Case Study Treatment Plan Sheet

Page 2

Case Study (Client Name; Dx.): *Ida; Right Humeral Fracture, 6 days post*

Group Members' Names: _____

Short-Term Goals	Methods	Rationale	Tx Approach/ Frame of Reference	Specific Activity/ Modality

Chapter

6

Ida

Teacher with a Right Humeral Fracture, 6 Weeks Postoperative

PART 1

Ida is a 55-year-old female referred to outpatient OT on November 25th s/p right humeral fracture. Ida is an elementary school teacher. She fell at school on October 14th. She lives with her husband who is retired. The physician has ordered OT evaluation and treatment.

TUTORIAL SESSION SHEET

Case Study (Pt. Name, Dx.): Ida; Right Humeral Fracture, 6 weeks post

Group Members' Names: _____

Facts/Knowledge

What do you already know that will help you to approach this case?

1. Individual client—roles, tasks, activities
2. The client's physical/sociocultural environment
3. Clinical signs and symptoms, treatment for diagnosis

Learning Issues

What questions do you need to ask to learn about:

1. Individual client—roles, tasks, activities
2. The client's physical/sociocultural environment
3. Clinical signs and symptoms, treatment for diagnosis

Actions/Steps to Learn

What are the plans to find the answers to your questions?

Part 2

Ida has been in excellent health. She has had no significant health problems. Ida fractured her humerus at the mid-humeral level. There was no surgical procedure. Initially, the physician immobilized her RUE in a sling and swathe. The physician is allowing her to do all light ADL and home chores but cautioned her about lifting anything heavy with the right arm. After a 2 week absence, Ida returned to work and is managing most aspects of her job (primarily paperwork) although she complains of writing fatigue. She occasionally needs help from co-workers to reach, lift, and carry needed items.

CASE STUDY EVALUATION PLAN

Case Study (Pt. Name, Dx.): Ida; Right Humeral Fracture, 6 weeks post

Group Members' Names: _____

Concerns/Performance Components/Areas	Assessments	How will assessment results be used?

PART 3

Ida is able to bathe and dress herself and perform all grooming activities, although she says she needs extra time to perform these activities and struggles at times because she is predominately using her nondominant left hand. She is independent in all transfers. She is doing light cooking. She is also doing laundry and light cleaning with her husband's assistance.

Ida complains of a minimal amount of pain in her right upper arm when attempting to reach for an object. She rates the pain level as a 5 on a scale of 1 to 10. Ida has minimal edema in the right hand. Her grip strength in her right hand is 7 pounds compared to 25 pounds in the left hand as measured by the dynamometer. AROM in the right wrist and finger motions is WFL. AROM in right shoulder flexion and abduction is 0 to 60 degrees, and in external rotation it is 0 to 20 degrees. AROM in the right elbow is 5 degrees to 115 degrees. Sensation for light touch is intact throughout the RUE. The strength and AROM in Ida's left arm is WFL. The physician has ordered AROM, mild resistive exercises, and ADL training. What will you do to help Ida?

In order to use a client-centered approach, select one person in your group to "be" Ida. This person can then tell you more about her roles, tasks, activities, interests, and priorities (this can be pretend) to assist you in developing your treatment plan and selecting appropriate therapeutic activities.

CASE STUDY TREATMENT PLAN SHEET

Page 1

Case Study (Client Name; Dx.): Ida; Right Humeral Fracture, 6 weeks post

Group Members' Names: _____

Deficits	Stage-Specific Cause	Short-Term Goals	Relates to which deficit	Functional Outcomes	Relates to which STG

CASE STUDY TREATMENT PLAN SHEET

Case Study (Client Name; Dx.): Ida; Right Humeral Fracture, 6 weeks post

Group Members' Names: _____

Short-Term Goals	Methods	Rationale	Tx Approach/ Frame of Reference	Specific Activity/ Modality

Chapter

Betty

Homemaker with a Left Colles Fracture; ORIF of the Left Hip

PART 1

Betty is a 56-year-old female who was admitted to the Hard Work Rehabilitation Hospital and was referred to OT on February 3rd. Her diagnosis is left Colles fracture and ORIF of the left hip. Betty fell in the parking lot of her condominium on January 28th. The physician has ordered occupational therapy to evaluate and treat.

TUTORIAL SESSION SHEET

Case Study (Pt. Name, Dx.): Betty; Left Colles Fracture; ORIF of Left Hip

Group Members' Names: _____

Facts/Knowledge	Learning Issues	Actions/Steps to Learn
What do you already know that will help you to approach this case?	What questions do you need to ask to learn about:	What are the plans to find the answers to your questions?
1. Individual client—roles, tasks, activities	1. Individual client—roles, tasks, activities	
2. The client's physical/sociocultural environment	2. The client's physical/sociocultural environment	
3. Clinical signs and symptoms, treatment for diagnosis	3. Clinical signs and symptoms, treatment for diagnosis	

PART 2

On Betty's first visit to see you, you interview her and find out the following information. Betty has been in excellent health prior to this injury. She lives with her husband Barney, her 76-year-old mother, and her dog. Betty states that she was walking her dog in the parking lot when a cat attacked her. She tripped over the curb trying to get away. Betty's husband has a left below knee amputation secondary to peripheral vascular disease and diabetes. Her mother is capable of performing her own self-care but not capable of instrumental ADL. Betty had been very active in her local amputee support group prior to her injury. She frequently would drive members to their medical appointments. Betty is anxious about her present situation because she is left-handed and states she is not able to do very much for herself.

In the emergency room on January 28th, the emergency room physician performed a closed reduction and applied a plaster cast from midhumeral level to the MP joints of the hand. The elbow was casted in approximately 90 degrees of elbow flexion and the wrist was casted in neutral position. You note that the left digits are swollen. She had surgery for an ORIF of the left femur secondary to a fracture of the femoral neck.

CASE STUDY EVALUATION PLAN

Case Study (Pt. Name, Dx.): Betty; Left Colles Fracture; ORIF of Left Hip

Group Members' Names: _____

Concerns/Performance Components/Areas	Assessments	How will assessment results be used?

PART 3

You have evaluated Betty and have found the following.

Betty tells you she is concerned about her husband and her mother. She states that they do the cooking and the housework. At the present time, her sister-in-law, who lives in the same town, visits frequently to prepare meals and provide other assistance as needed. She is angry at herself for letting a cat get the best of her.

Betty c/o moderate pain in her left upper extremity, mainly the wrist and fingers. She rates her pain as a 6 on a scale of 1 to 10. Severe edema is noted in all of the digits of the left hand (approximately two times the size of the right hand). She has a great deal of difficulty flexing her fingers to make a fist (the cast restricts the MP motion). She is unable to oppose her thumb to any finger. She is unable to hold any objects in her left hand because of the cast. She states that at times her hand feels numb and other times she has paresthesia. Sensation for light touch is intact in areas of the LUE not covered by the cast.

Betty's physical therapist tells you that she will be using a platform walker and that the physician has restricted her to partial weightbearing (PWB) on the LLE. Presently she is requiring moderate assistance with stand pivot transfers from the bed to the bedside commode and minimal assistance with sit to stand transfers. She requires minimal assistance to move from side sit to supine in bed.

Betty is unable to don some types of blouses and dresses over the cast and is not able to don pants or skirts with closures. She requires moderate assistance to don underpants and socks. She is unable to don her bra, socks, or tie shoes/sneakers. Because of the inability to use her dominant left hand, Betty is unable to manage buttons, has difficulty feeding herself with her nondominant right hand, she spills food on herself frequently. She also requires minimal assistance with personal hygiene after toileting, and requires moderate assistance with sponge bathing. She requires minimal assistance to brush her teeth. She is dependent in simple meal preparation and other household chores such as cleaning.

Betty tells you it is very important for her to be able to care for herself (grooming, bathing, and dressing). She is really looking forward to being able to get in her shower to bathe when she goes home. She also wants to be able to prepare meals for herself, her husband, and her mother.

Betty will probably be in the rehabilitation hospital for 4 weeks. What will you do to help Betty?

In order to use a client-centered approach, select one person in your group to "be" Betty. This person can then tell you more about her roles, tasks, activities, interests, and priorities (this can be "pretend") to assist you in developing your treatment plan and selecting appropriate therapeutic activities.

CASE STUDY TREATMENT PLAN SHEET

Case Study (Client Name; Dx.): Betty; Left Colles Fracture; ORIF of Left Hip

Group Members' Names: _____

Page 1

Deficits	Stage-Specific Cause	Short-Term Goals	Relates to which deficit	Functional Outcomes	Relates to which STG

CASE STUDY TREATMENT PLAN SHEET

Case Study (Client Name; Dx.): Betty; Left Colles Fracture; ORIF of Left Hip

Group Members' Names: _____

Short-Term Goals	Methods	Rationale	Tx Approach/ Frame of Reference	Specific Activity/ Modality

Chapter

Esther

Retired Office Manager with a Right Total Hip Replacement

PART 1

Esther is an 86-year-old female who was referred to home health OT on March 23rd. Esther fractured her right hip on March 3rd and had a right total hip replacement (THR) on March 4th. The physician has ordered OT to evaluate and treat.

You call to make arrangements to see Esther. She answers the phone and seems anxious about being able to manage her daily living tasks. She is cognitively intact and gives you excellent directions on how to get to her condominium.

TUTORIAL SESSION SHEET

Case Study (Pt. Name, Dx.): Esther; Right Total Hip Replacement

Group Members' Names: _____

Facts/Knowledge	Learning Issues	Actions/Steps to Learn
What do you already know that will help you to approach this case?	What questions do you need to ask to learn about:	What are the plans to find the answers to your questions?
1. Individual client—roles, tasks, activities	1. Individual client—roles, tasks, activities	
2. The client's physical/sociocultural environment	2. The client's physical/sociocultural environment	
3. Clinical signs and symptoms, treatment for diagnosis	3. Clinical signs and symptoms, treatment for diagnosis	

PART 2

On your first visit to see Esther, you interview her and find out the following information. Esther has been in excellent health prior to this injury. She is a widow who lives alone in a second floor condominium. The elevator is 50 feet down the catwalk from her front door.

Esther states that she fell in the kitchen late one evening. A neighbor found her there the next morning. Esther tells you the doctor wasn't sure if she fell because her hip fractured or she fractured her hip because she fell. Esther had 2 weeks of physical therapy before being discharged home. She is weightbearing as tolerated (WBAT).

CASE STUDY EVALUATION PLAN

Case Study (Pt. Name, Dx.): Esther; Right Total Hip Replacement

Group Members' Names: _____

Concerns/Performance Components/Areas	Assessments	How will assessment results be used?

PART 3

Esther has a home health aide coming to help her with her self-care activities but she wants very badly to do these tasks independently. She requires maximal assistance with lower body self-care. Since getting home she has just been wearing a housecoat and slippers. She tells you that she took a "cat bath" on the day the home health aide didn't come, but she would love to be able to get in and out of her bathtub. Presently, she is unable to lift her right leg over the edge of the bathtub due to weakness.

Esther is able to use her walker independently to move around her condominium, but finds it difficult to carry things while using the walker. She has a raised toilet seat and is able to transfer on and off independently. She states that she has some difficulty getting into bed at night.

Esther prides herself on her independence and is especially proud of her home cooking. Having always cooked for herself, she states she is not eating very well because she is unable to get to the grocery store to buy groceries. She doesn't drive and has relied on the city bus to take her to the grocery store and doctor's office since her husband's passing last year. Esther has no immediate family in the area. She has a neighbor who has brought her a few meals, however, she is a very proud woman and has difficulty asking for help from her neighbors.

Esther is also concerned about being able to keep her condominium in sparkling condition. She asks you if the home health aide can take out her garbage and clean her condominium for her.

What will you do to help Esther?

In order to use a client-centered approach, select one person in your group to "be" Esther. This person can then tell you more about her roles, tasks, activities, interests, and priorities to assist you in developing your treatment plan and selecting appropriate therapeutic activities.

CASE STUDY TREATMENT PLAN SHEET

Page 1

Case Study (Client Name; Dx.): *Esther; Right Total Hip Replacement*

Group Members' Names: _____

Deficits	Stage-Specific Cause	Short-Term Goals	Relates to which deficit	Functional Outcomes	Relates to which STG

CASE STUDY TREATMENT PLAN SHEET

Page 2

Case Study (Client Name; Dx.): Esther; Right Total Hip Replacement

Group Members' Names: _____

Short-Term Goals	Methods	Rationale	Tx Approach/ Frame of Reference	Specific Activity/ Modality

Chapter

Mary

Clerical Worker with Acute Exacerbation of Rheumatoid Arthritis

PART 1

Mary is a 31-year-old female referred to home health OT on August 8th with a diagnosis of acute exacerbation of rheumatoid arthritis (RA). Mary was first diagnosed with RA 6 years ago. The physician has ordered OT to evaluate and treat.

TUTORIAL SESSION SHEET

Case Study (Pt. Name, Dx.): Mary; Acute Exacerbation of Rheumatoid Arthritis

Group Members' Names: _____

Facts/Knowledge	Learning Issues	Actions/Steps to Learn
What do you already know that will help you to approach this case? 1. Individual client—roles, tasks, activities 2. The client's physical/sociocultural environment 3. Clinical signs and symptoms, treatment for diagnosis	What questions do you need to ask to learn about: 1. Individual client—roles, tasks, activities 2. The client's physical/sociocultural environment 3. Clinical signs and symptoms, treatment for diagnosis	What are the plans to find the answers to your questions?

PART 2

On Mary's first visit you interview her and find out the following information. Mary has had minimal medical problems other than the RA. She lives with her two children, a girl age 11 and a boy age 8, and her significant other. She has difficulty managing her children. They tease her about her disability. Mary worked in the town hall as a clerk up until 3 months ago when she was placed on disability due to the arthritis. Her significant other is supportive. He owns his own plumbing supply business and is able to take time off of work as needed. He drives her to medical appointments, shopping, or wherever she wants to go, because she no longer drives. Mary is very anxious about her present situation because she is right-handed and states she is not able to do very much for herself. She feels that she is becoming more and more dependent. She has not had OT before.

CASE STUDY EVALUATION PLAN

Case Study (Pt. Name, Dx.): Mary; Acute Exacerbation of Rheumatoid Arthritis

Group Members' Names: _____

Concerns/Performance Components/Areas	Assessments	How will assessment results be used?

PART 3

You have evaluated Mary and have found the following.

Mary is depressed about her functional limitations. Mary is right hand dominant. She has swollen, inflamed joints bilaterally in the elbows, wrists, all MP joints and interphalangeal (IP) joints. Moderate edema is noted in hands bilaterally. She has ulnar drift bilaterally at MP joints in both hands (digits deviated ulnarly 10 degrees from midline). AROM measures (physician has approved AROM exercises) as follows. Bilateral wrist extension 0 to 40 degrees; bilateral wrist flexion 0 to 35 degrees; bilateral radial deviation of the wrist is 0 to 10 degrees; bilateral ulnar deviation of the wrist is 0 to 15 degrees; MP flexion (all joints) 0 to 75 degrees; IP flexion (all joints) 0 to 85 degrees; bilateral elbow flexion extension 10 to 95 degrees. Mary's shoulder joints are not presently inflamed but she has pain on movement and crepitus is noted. The following AROM deficits are noted: right shoulder flexion 0 to 100 degrees; left shoulder flexion 0 to 95 degrees; right shoulder abduction 0 to 90 degrees; left shoulder abduction 0 to 85 degrees; bilateral external rotation 0 to 35 degrees; bilateral internal rotation 0 to 50 degrees.

Mary also complains of pain in both hips, knees, and ankles, limiting her walking ability. She tires after approximately 200 feet due to the pain.

Mary complains of paresthesia in both hands and numbness in the fingertips. She has limited ability to use her hands for functional activities. She is presently unable to manage buttons, zippers, and snaps on her clothing. She requires excess time to tie her sneakers. She is unable to don or doff panty hose due to inability to reach to her feet. She also needs someone to hook her bra in the back. She has a great deal of difficulty getting in and out of the bottom of the bathtub to baths and is taking sponge baths since her exacerbation. This is even difficult as she frequently drops the soap and the washcloth. Her daughter puts toothpaste on her toothbrush for her. She has difficulty managing the toothbrush and frequently drops it. She no longer flosses as she can't hold the thin floss.

Mary loves to cook but now is unable to open jars, cans, food boxes, milk cartons, or other containers. She is only able to lift lightweight pots and even then has pain when doing so. Cutting food has been very painful for her hands. Her daughter has been doing the housecleaning for the last year but very reluctantly. Mary would like to do more but the pain limits her ability and her endurance.

You notice the watercolor paintings that Mary painted in recent years hanging on the wall. She has stopped painting because she can't hold the paint brushes nor manage the paint containers.

What will you do to help Mary?

In order to use a client-centered approach, select one person in your group to "be" Mary. This person can then tell you more about her roles, tasks, activities, interests, and priorities to assist you in developing your treatment plan and selecting appropriate therapeutic activities.

CASE STUDY TREATMENT PLAN SHEET

Page 1

Case Study (Client Name; Dx.): Mary; Acute Exacerbation of Rheumatoid Arthritis

Group Members' Names: _____

Deficits	Stage-Specific Cause	Short-Term Goals	Relates to which deficit	Functional Outcomes	Relates to which STG

CASE STUDY TREATMENT PLAN SHEET

Case Study (Client Name; Dx.): Mary; Acute Exacerbation of Rheumatoid Arthritis

Group Members' Names: _____

Short-Term Goals	Methods	Rationale	Tx Approach/ Frame of Reference	Specific Activity/ Modality

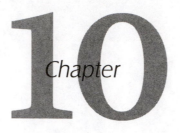

Chapter

10

Susie

Butcher's Assistant with Scleroderma

PART 1

Susie is a 45-year-old female referred to outpatient OT on October 26th with a diagnosis of scleroderma (dSSc). Her physician has ordered OT to evaluate and treat.

TUTORIAL SESSION SHEET

Case Study (Pt. Name, Dx.): Susie; Scleroderma

Group Members' Names: _____

Facts/Knowledge

What do you already know that will help you to approach this case?

1. Individual client—roles, tasks, activities
2. The client's physical/sociocultural environment
3. Clinical signs and symptoms, treatment for diagnosis

Learning Issues

What questions do you need to ask to learn about:

1. Individual client—roles, tasks, activities
2. The client's physical/sociocultural environment
3. Clinical signs and symptoms, treatment for diagnosis

Actions/Steps to Learn

What are the plans to find the answers to your questions?

PART 2

On Susie's first visit, you interview her and find out the following information. Susie has complained of her hands being cold and fingers being tight for the last year or so. She lives alone with her cat and her dog. She is divorced with no children. Her elderly parents live in Michigan. Susie loves to play bingo. A great evening to her is to go to the bingo hall with her markers, her lucky charms, and a pack of Marlboros. She went to the doctor when she began to experience pain in her finger-tips when playing bingo, causing her to drop the markers frequently.

Susie tells you she works at the local supermarket in the meat department. She thought her hands were always cold because of her frequent trips to the meat locker and working in a cold room. She says her hands often ache and she is barely able to make a fist. She states that she gets tired more quickly at work and her ankles feel "tight." She thought this was because she was just getting older. Susie also tells you that she owns her own home and does her own yard work, including mowing the lawn and tending to her flowerbeds in which she takes great pride. She states she also loves to cook. She usually cooks most of the day on Sunday and then eats leftovers for most of the week.

CASE STUDY EVALUATION PLAN

Case Study (Pt. Name, Dx.): Susie; Scleroderma

Group Members' Names: _____

Concerns/Performance Components/Areas	Assessments	How will assessment results be used?

PART 3

You look at her hands and note mild to moderate edema in both hands. She has an open sore on the second and third IP joints of the right hand and the second IP joint on the left hand. Susie tells you she is right-handed. You measure range of motion. A/PROM measurements are as follows: Bilateral MP joints—(1st, 0 to 45), (2nd, 0 to 75), (3rd, 0 to 80), (4th, 0 to 75), (5th, 0 to 85). Bilateral IP joints—(1st, 0 to 60), (2nd, 5 to 100), (3rd, 10 to 95), (4th, 10 to 95), (5th, 5 to 100). There appears to be shortening of the thumb web space bilaterally and in finger abduction. You measure grip strength. Her right hand measures 16 pounds and the left measures 12 pounds. Three point pinch is 4 pounds in the right and 3 pounds in the left. Lateral pinch is 8 pounds in the right and 6 pounds in the left. What will you do to help Susie?

In order to use a client-centered approach, select one person in your group to "be" Susie. This person can then tell you about her roles, tasks, activities, interests, and priorities to assist you in developing your treatment plan and selecting appropriate therapeutic activities.

CASE STUDY TREATMENT PLAN SHEET

Page 1

Case Study (Client Name; Dx.): Susie; Scleroderma

Group Members' Names: _____

Deficits	Stage Specific Cause	Short-Term Goals	Relates to which deficit	Functional Outcomes	Relates to which STG

CASE STUDY TREATMENT PLAN SHEET

Case Study (Client Name; Dx.): Susie; Scleroderma

Group Members' Names: _____

Short-Term Goals	Methods	Rationale	Tx Approach/ Frame of Reference	Specific Activity/ Modality

11

Iva

Homemaker and Mail Clerk with Chronic Rheumatoid Arthritis

This case study consists of one part only. You may use the Tutorial Session Sheet to help guide your learning. Use the Case Study Treatment Plan Sheet to develop a treatment plan.

CASE STUDY

Iva is a 34-year-old female referred to outpatient OT with a diagnosis of chronic RA. Iva was first diagnosed when she was 19 years old. The physician has ordered OT to evaluate and treat.

On Iva's first visit you interview her and find out the following information. Iva is cognitively intact. She reports that she has had minimal medical problems other than the RA. She lives with her husband and her daughter, a girl age 11. Her daughter is very helpful to her mother but Iva feels this is taking away from her daughter's childhood.

Iva works part-time as a mail clerk for American Express. Her husband is a computer salesman. He frequently travels to attend trade shows. Iva's husband is the primary driver in the family, but Iva will drive if she has to. Iva is very anxious about her present situation because she is in a great deal of pain and has difficulty with her self-care, homemaking, and work tasks. She feels that she is becoming more and more dependent.

Iva reports that she is depressed about her inability to use her hands in functional activities. Iva is right hand dominant. She presently has a great deal of pain and difficulty managing buttons, zippers, and snaps on her clothing. She requires excess time to tie her sneakers. She also has difficulty donning and doffing panty hose and her bra.

Iva loves to take a hot shower in the morning to loosen up, however, she complains that it is even get-ting difficult to stand for that length of time in the shower stall. Holding and manipulating grooming aids such as a toothbrush, hairbrush, and make-up is increasingly difficult because of pain in her hands. Luckily, Iva's daughter helps her with meal preparation by opening containers, lifting heavy containers, and cutting foods. These tasks also had caused pain in Iva's hands.

Iva also complains of pain in both hips, knees, and ankles, limiting her walking ability. She tires after approximately 200 feet due to the pain. Iva also states that it has become increasingly difficult to do her job due to the pain in her knees and her limited walking ability. Iva's job requires her to sort the mail and then deliver the mail to various departments. The building is very large. It takes her close to 3 hours to walk the entire building delivering the mail. She stops to rest frequently because of the pain.

She has swollen, inflamed joints and moderately decreased AROM bilaterally in the elbows, wrists, MP joints, and IP joints. She has ulnar drift bilaterally at MP joints in both hands—deviated ulnarly 10 degrees from midline. In addition, Iva complains of paresthesia in both hands and numbness in the fingertips. Iva's shoulder joints are not presently inflamed but she has pain on movement and crepitus is noted. Due to her pain, Iva demonstrates moderate deficits in bilateral shoulder AROM (unable to reach behind her head or back; unable to reach up or out above shoulder level). What will you do to help Iva?

In order to use a client-centered approach, select one person in your group to "be" Iva. This person can then tell you about her roles, tasks, activities, interests, and priorities to assist you in developing your treatment plan and selecting appropriate therapeutic activities.

TUTORIAL SESSION SHEET

Case Study (Pt. Name, Dx.): Iva; Chronic Rheumatoid Arthritis

Group Members' Names: _____

Facts/Knowledge

What do you already know that will help you to approach this case?

1. Individual client—roles, tasks, activities
2. The client's physical/sociocultural environment
3. Clinical signs and symptoms, treatment for diagnosis

Learning Issues

What questions do you need to ask to learn about:

1. Individual client—roles, tasks, activities
2. The client's physical/sociocultural environment
3. Clinical signs and symptoms, treatment for diagnosis

Actions/Steps to Learn

What are the plans to find the answers to your questions?

CASE STUDY TREATMENT PLAN SHEET

Page 1

Case Study (Client Name; Dx.): *Iva; Chronic Rheumatoid Arthritis*

Group Members' Names: _____

Deficits	Stage-Specific Cause	Short-Term Goals	Relates to which deficit	Functional Outcomes	Relates to which STG

CASE STUDY TREATMENT PLAN SHEET

Page 2

Case Study (Client Name; Dx.): Iva; Chronic Rheumatoid Arthritis

Group Members' Names: _____

Short-Term Goals	Methods	Rationale	Tx Approach/ Frame of Reference	Specific Activity/ Modality

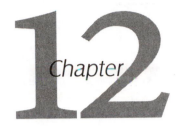

Chapter 12

Doris

Teacher with Systemic Lupus Erythematosus

Case study developed by Barbara L. Kornblau, JD, OTR/L, FAOTA, DAAPM, ABDA, CDMS, CCM

Doris, age 34, works as a teacher for the Anderson County public schools. For about 2 years, she has had difficulty with joint pain and hot flashes during which her blood pressure changes rapidly. After 2 years of complaining, she is finally diagnosed with lupus. She is referred to you by her physician for treatment, patient education, and management of her symptoms. You work in an outpatient clinic. Doris' medical insurance policy will cover any OT services that you recommend.

The doctor has told her to avoid exposure to the light because of the lupus which is causing the hot flashes and blood pressure fluctuation. She tells you that as a teacher she is expected to take her students out to the playground from 1:00 until 1:45, when the sun is at its strongest. Also, her classroom is located on the side of the building that gets the afternoon sun.

The joints in her hands have become extremely inflamed. She is having difficulty writing and filling out forms such as report cards. Even typing on the computer causes joint pain occasionally. She also has difficulty carrying books and supplies from the office and storerooms to her classroom.

After 2 years of complaining without a real diagnosis, Doris' principal thinks she is a hypochondriac. Up until now, any time Doris asked for assistance, he shrugged his shoulders and told her to try a little harder. His famous line has become, "There are no special privileges in this world."

Doris has been out on sick leave for 1 week following discharge from the hospital where the diagnosis of lupus was finally made. She knows she will have to return to work shortly and is scared to death of returning to her job. She knows there will need to be some changes at work in order for her to continue to perform her job, but she doesn't know what changes she needs or how to approach her principal about making those changes.

What will you do to help Doris?

In order to use a client-centered approach, select one person in your group to "be" Doris. This person can then tell you about her roles, tasks, activities, interests, and priorities to assist you in developing your treatment plan and selecting appropriate therapeutic activities.

TUTORIAL SESSION SHEET

Case Study (Pt. Name, Dx.): Doris; Systemic Lupus Erythematosus (SLE)

Group Members' Names: _____

Facts/Knowledge

What do you already know that will help you to approach this case?

1. Individual client—roles, tasks, activities
2. The client's physical/sociocultural environment
3. Clinical signs and symptoms, treatment for diagnosis

Learning Issues

What questions do you need to ask to learn about:

1. Individual client—roles, tasks, activities
2. The client's physical/sociocultural environment
3. Clinical signs and symptoms, treatment for diagnosis

Actions/Steps to Learn

What are the plans to find the answers to your questions?

CASE STUDY TREATMENT PLAN SHEET

Page 1

Case Study (Client Name; Dx.): *Doris; Systemic Lupus Erythematosus (SLE)*

Group Members' Names: _____

Deficits	Stage-Specific Cause	Short-Term Goals	Relates to which deficit	Functional Outcomes	Relates to which STG

CASE STUDY TREATMENT PLAN SHEET

Page 2

Case Study (Client Name; Dx.): Doris; Systemic Lupus Erythematosus (SLE)

Group Members' Names: _____

Short-Term Goals	Methods	Rationale	Tx Approach/ Frame of Reference	Specific Activity/ Modality

13

Frank

Power Company Lineman with a Right Below Elbow Amputation, 4 Days Postoperative

Frank is a 27-year-old who was referred to inpatient OT on February 8th with a diagnosis of below elbow amputation of the RUE. Frank was working as a lineman for National Power and Light (NPL) when he was hit with a backfeed of 5000 volts of electricity. This injury required amputation of the RUE at the mid forearm level. This accident occurred on February 4th. The physician has ordered OT to evaluate and treat. Frank is scheduled for discharge in about a week or 2 and will then continue as an outpatient. Planning long-term, the physician has also asked for your opinion on the type of prosthesis to order for Frank.

During Frank's first therapy session, you interview him and find out the following information. Frank is right hand dominant. Frank has a previous history of a fractured left shoulder suffered in a fall 3 years ago when working on the lines. Otherwise, he has been in excellent health. Frank has been employed by NPL for 7 years. NPL provides excellent medical coverage for their employees. Your inpatient facility has an outpatient department, so you will be able to see Frank through the course of his rehabilitation. Frank is single and considers himself a real ladies man. His present girlfriend works as a registered nurse in a local hospital. He is reluctant to leave his hospital room as he feels people are always looking at him because of the obvious amputation. His friends have been supportive and come by to visit frequently.

Frank requires assistance to manage clothes closures—buttons, zippers, belt, shoelaces—secondary to only having use of the nondominant left hand. He also requires minimal assistance to don a button down shirt, pullover shirt, pants, socks, and shoes. He is able to shave using an electric razor in his left hand. He is able to brush his teeth using one-handed techniques. Frank is able to feed himself with his left hand although he still spills food at times and he needs his girlfriend to cut his food and butter his toast. Frank used to prepare himself simple meals at home but is very concerned that he will no longer be able to do this because he is unable to use both hands.

He is very concerned about his ability to continue to work in some capacity. Prior to his accident, Frank was enrolled in a computer science program at a local community college because he wished to change careers to information technology and web development. He is afraid that he will not be able to continue with classes as "he cannot take notes or write the papers." He states that it is very difficult to type on the computer or use the computer mouse.

Frank is also concerned about "getting out of shape." Prior to the accident Frank spent much of his free time at a local gym.

Frank's stump is healing well. He does experience phantom sensation and his stump is hypersensitive. Sensation for light touch is impaired at the very distal end of the stump. The stump is bulbous and has minimal scarring. AROM of the elbow is WNL. Strength of the remaining musculature is as follows:

- Forearm pronators and supinators—fair plus
- Elbow flexors—good minus
- Elbow extensors—good

All other muscle groups in the RUE are WNL and ROM and strength in the LUE are WNL.

What will you do to help Frank?

In order to use a client-centered approach, select one person in your group to "be" Frank. This person can then tell you about his roles, tasks, activities, interests, and priorities to assist you in developing your treatment plan and selecting appropriate therapeutic activities.

TUTORIAL SESSION SHEET

Case Study (Pt. Name, Dx.): Frank; Right Below Elbow Amputation, 4 days post

Group Members' Names:

Facts/Knowledge	Learning Issues	Actions/Steps to Learn
What do you already know that will help you to approach this case? 1. Individual client—roles, tasks, activities 2. The client's physical/sociocultural environment 3. Clinical signs and symptoms, treatment for diagnosis	What questions do you need to ask to learn about: 1. Individual client—roles, tasks, activities 2. The client's physical/sociocultural environment 3. Clinical signs and symptoms, treatment for diagnosis	What are the plans to find the answers to your questions?

Case Study Treatment Plan Sheet

Page 1

Case Study (Client Name; Dx.): Frank; Right Below Elbow Amputation, 4 days post

Group Members' Names: _____

Deficits	Stage-Specific Cause	Short-Term Goals	Relates to which deficit	Functional Outcomes	Relates to which STG

Case Study Treatment Plan Sheet

Page 2

Case Study (Client Name; Dx.): *Frank; Right Below Elbow Amputation, 4 days post*

Group Members' Names: _____

Short-Term Goals	Methods	Rationale	Tx Approach/ Frame of Reference	Specific Activity/ Modality

Chapter 14

James

Actor with a Right Below Knee Amputation, 5 Days Postoperative

James is a 28-year-old referred to inpatient OT in a rehabilitation hospital on September 20, with a diagnosis of below knee amputation of the right lower extremity (RLE). James suffered traumatic injuries to his right leg in a motorcycle accident requiring the amputation. This accident occurred on September 15th.

James is single. He is a real risk taker in the types of activities he likes. Skiing, parasailing, kayaking, and mountain climbing are among his favorites. He works as an actor in the motion picture industry. He is very concerned about his ability to continue to work in some capacity as appearance is very important in the motion picture industry.

James is very gregarious. He states that he wants to get out as soon as possible and drive his Ferrari again. He loves going down to the local bar to meet with other young actors. He also loves to escort several young actresses to Hollywood parties, but fears no actress will want to go out with him.

In the hospital, the nurses bring all his grooming supplies to his bed and he is able to brush his teeth, shave with an electric razor, and comb his hair. He requires minimal assistance to move from supine to side sit on the edge of the bed. He needs moderate to maximal assistance to don and doff his pants in bed. He presently requires moderate assistance with transfers from bed to bedside commode and from bed to wheelchair. He has only taken bed baths. He can't imagine how he will get into his bathtub at home. James has a bathtub with Jacuzzi jets. James states his plan is to return to his luxury apartment with help 24 hours a day, as he is expecting a big settlement as a result of the accident. All rooms in his apartment are accessible except for the bathroom.

James is able to ambulate 50 feet with crutches. He feels he is too slow. James is independent in using the wheelchair provided by the rehabilitation hospital, but complains that he sometimes feels like the chair will tip over. He also wants to get power wheelchair "for going out and going fast." James states he has "not worked out how to get the power chair into his Ferrari."

James' stump is healing well. He states he is experiencing phantom sensation and hypersensitivity in the RLE. The stump is bulbous. The prosthetist is presently working with James to fit him with a temporary prosthesis. James will continue as an outpatient after discharge from the hospital.

What will you do to help James?

In order to use a client-centered approach, select one person in your group to "be" James. This person can then tell you about his roles, tasks, activities, interests, and priorities to assist you in developing your treatment plan and selecting appropriate therapeutic activities.

TUTORIAL SESSION SHEET

Case Study (Pt. Name, Dx.): James; Right Below Knee Amputation, 5 days post

Group Members' Names: _____

Facts/Knowledge	Learning Issues	Actions/Steps to Learn
What do you already know that will help you to approach this case?	What questions do you need to ask to learn about:	What are the plans to find the answers to your questions?
1. Individual client—roles, tasks, activities	1. Individual client—roles, tasks, activities	
2. The client's physical/sociocultural environment	2. The client's physical/sociocultural environment	
3. Clinical signs and symptoms, treatment for diagnosis	3. Clinical signs and symptoms, treatment for diagnosis	

CASE STUDY TREATMENT PLAN SHEET

Page 1

Case Study (Client Name; Dx.): James; Right Below Knee Amputation, 5 days post

Group Members' Names: _____

Deficits	Stage-Specific Cause	Short-Term Goals	Relates to which deficit	Functional Outcomes	Relates to which STG

Case Study Treatment Plan Sheet

Case Study (Client Name; Dx.): *James; Right Below Knee Amputation, 5 days post*

Group Members' Names: _____

Short-Term Goals	Methods	Rationale	Tx Approach/ Frame of Reference	Specific Activity/ Modality

Chapter 15

Barney

Insurance Salesman with a Left Below Knee and Right Above Knee Amputations

Barney is a 57-year-old male referred to OT in a general hospital that has both acute care and a rehabilitation unit. Barney just had surgery for a left below knee amputation 2 days ago. He had a right above knee amputation 3 years ago. His physician has ordered OT to evaluate and treat.

On reviewing Barney's medical chart you find that he has peripheral vascular disease, has insulin-dependent diabetes mellitus (IDDM), and has peripheral neuropathy. You also find out that he lives with his elderly mother-in-law and his wife in a second floor condominium. Three months ago his wife was attacked by a cat and she fractured her left wrist and left hip. She is home now and progressing well but still uses a straight cane to get around. Barney and his wife Betty had hired a day housekeeper to help them at home with cooking, general housework, and taking care of his elderly mother. About 6 months before his second amputation, Barney was independent in all his self-care, independent in simple meal preparation tasks, and would drive his mother-in-law to the doctor's office as needed. Betty was concerned about him driving because his vision was failing, and he seemed to have "increasing nervousness in his hands." This "nervousness" caused him some difficulty with feeding himself because the food would occasionally fall off of the spoon. He was also beginning to have difficulty with writing.

The rehabilitation aide brings Barney to the rehabilitation unit for you to evaluate his status. Barney is pleasant, alert, and oriented x 3. His long- and short-term memory are intact. Barney is a financial planner and works from his office at home. His secretary/assistant is presently managing his insurance business under his direction. Prior to this amputation, Barney was getting around his apartment using his prosthesis and a walker. He states that he has a "clunker" of a wheelchair. He uses it very rarely when going out because it is very heavy to load in the car and very difficult to maneuver. He is not sure how easy it will be to manage a wheelchair in his home or his home office. He is very concerned about how he, his wife, and mother-in-law are going to manage.

His static sitting balance is fair to good. He is unable to take more than a minimal challenge to his sitting balance. His UE strength is in fair plus range throughout. You note a mild tremor in both hands. Fine motor coordination is fair and sensation for light touch and proprioception is impaired in both UEs, especially the hands. He presently requires a two man lift from bed to bedside commode and from bed to wheelchair. He requires minimal assistance to move from supine to side sit on the edge of the bed. Barney is embarrassed because he requires maximal assistance with cleaning himself after using the bedside commode.

Barney is able to don a pullover shirt but needs assistance with buttoning a button down shirt. He needs moderate to maximal assistance to don and doff his pants in bed. In the hospital, the nurses bring all his grooming supplies to his bed and he is able to brush his teeth, shave with an electric razor, and comb his hair. He has been taking bed baths. He wants to be able to get into his bathtub once he gets home. Before this amputation, he would sit on the edge of the tub, remove his prosthesis and then lower himself to the bottom of the tub.

Barney will probably be in the rehabilitation unit for 1 month. He says he would probably get a prosthesis for his left leg, but his doctor says it will probably be more practical to use a wheelchair at home.

What will you do to help Barney?

In order to use a client-centered approach, select one person in your group to "be" Barney. This person can then tell you about his roles, tasks, activities, interests, and priorities to assist you in developing your treatment plan and selecting appropriate therapeutic activities.

TUTORIAL SESSION SHEET

Case Study (Pt. Name, Dx.): Barney; Left Below Knee and Right Above Knee Amputations

Group Members' Names: _____

Facts/Knowledge

What do you already know that will help you to approach this case?

1. Individual client—roles, tasks, activities
2. The client's physical/sociocultural environment
3. Clinical signs and symptoms, treatment for diagnosis

Learning Issues

What questions do you need to ask to learn about:

1. Individual client—roles, tasks, activities
2. The client's physical/sociocultural environment
3. Clinical signs and symptoms, treatment for diagnosis

Actions/Steps to Learn

What are the plans to find the answers to your questions?

CASE STUDY TREATMENT PLAN SHEET

Case Study (Client Name; Dx.): Barney; Left Below Knee and Right Above Knee Amputations

Group Members' Names: _____

Page 1

Deficits	Stage-Specific Cause	Short-Term Goals	Relates to which deficit	Functional Outcomes	Relates to which STG

Page 2

Case Study Treatment Plan Sheet

Case Study (Client Name; Dx.): Barney; Left Below Knee and Right Above Knee Amputations

Group Members' Names: _____

Short-Term Goals	Methods	Rationale	Tx Approach/ Frame of Reference	Specific Activity/ Modality

Chapter 16

Mark

Fireman with C6 Tetraplegia

Mark is a 30-year-old male who sustained complete C6 quadriplegia in a diving accident. Prior to his injury, Mark worked as a paid fireman. He also taught fire science part-time in the local community college and authored a textbook. He has been married for 5 years, he has no children despite trying for the past year. His wife is studying nursing in a local university. His hobbies include computers and photography. He has always been very independent, has a good sense of humor, and has a wide circle of friends. His parents and two brothers live in town and are very supportive. He has excellent health care insurance.

Mark was transferred to your rehabilitation facility. He is medically stable and surgical fusion has stabilized the fracture site. In reviewing the medical records, you note that strength in all innervated musculature is in good range. Sensory deficits follow the classical pattern for his level of spinal cord injury.

When you first meet Mark, he tells you he was shaken up the other day when all of a sudden he began sweating and had a terrific headache. The nurse helped him through this incident, explained that these symptoms might occur in people with high level spinal cord injuries. He knows she explained what to do when this happens, but he was so shaken that he cannot remember all the details.

Mark has not yet achieved maximum functional level for his level of spinal cord injury. He is particularly interested in being as independent as possible in all self-care activities. While he knows he won't be able to return to work as a fireman, he hopes to obtain some type of gainful employment. He is aware of adapted vehicles that might make it possible for him to drive. As he is very financially secure, he wants to modify his home to make it accessible.

Mark would also like to continue to participate in his hobbies. He says he has installed a voice activated system on his computer so he can use it for writing. He asks if his camera can be adapted because he would like to continue with photography.

What can you do to help Mark?

In order to use a client-centered approach, select one person in your group to "be" Mark. This person can then tell you about his roles, tasks, activities, interests, and priorities to assist you in developing your treatment plan and selecting appropriate therapeutic activities.

TUTORIAL SESSION SHEET

Case Study (Pt. Name, Dx.): Mark; C6 Tetraplegia

Group Members' Names: _____

Facts/Knowledge

What do you already know that will help you to approach this case?

1. Individual client—roles, tasks, activities
2. The client's physical/sociocultural environment
3. Clinical signs and symptoms, treatment for diagnosis

Learning Issues

What questions do you need to ask to learn about:

1. Individual client—roles, tasks, activities
2. The client's physical/sociocultural environment
3. Clinical signs and symptoms, treatment for diagnosis

Actions/Steps to Learn

What are the plans to find the answers to your questions?

CASE STUDY TREATMENT PLAN SHEET

Page 1

Case Study (Client Name; Dx.): Mark; C6 Tetraplegia

Group Members' Names: _____

Deficits	Stage-Specific Cause	Short Term Goals	Relates to which deficit	Functional Outcomes	Relates to which STG

Case Study Treatment Plan Sheet

Page 2

Case Study (Client Name; Dx.): Mark; C6 Tetraplegia

Group Members' Names: _____

Short-Term Goals	Methods	Rationale	Tx Approach/ Frame of Reference	Specific Activity/ Modality

George

High School Student with C5/C6 Tetraplegia

You are a therapist in a rehabilitation hospital. You have just finished your initial evaluation on George.

George is an 18-year-old male who has tetraplegia secondary to a football accident 1 week ago. George states that he was playing touch football when during one play a hard hit caused his neck to snap back. He recalls feeling shaken up and walking to the sidelines to sit out the next few plays. After approximately 5 minutes he began to experience numbness and inability to move his arms. His friends called an ambulance and he was taken to Our Lady of Notre Dame Hospital.

The physician has stated that George does not appear to have a severance of the spinal cord but there is severe edema around the cord. The prognosis at this point is guarded. George is to wear a cervical collar at all times. He is very fearful of movement and trusts very few people to help him in and out of bed into his reclining wheelchair.

George is concerned about his future. He had been planning to attend the University of Nebraska next year on a football scholarship. He is not a very good student and describes himself as motivated primarily by sports activities, photography, fishing, and ham radio operating. This is his senior year in high school. It is very important to him to graduate with the rest of his class. He knows that he will have to "buckle down" and work hard to do this, especially in view of this injury.

George states that he has many friends who call constantly to see how he is doing and to ask when he will be able to go out with them again. He enjoys their calls but feels "strange" when talking to friends because someone must hold the receiver and listens to the conversation. He wants to be able to use the phone independently, including making calls.

George has full PROM in both UE, he does however complain of pain at the end ROM in his right shoulder. Manual muscle test results are in Table 17-1.

Sensation for superficial pain, light touch, and temperature is absent below C5 level. He requires external support for sitting balance secondary to high level of injury. He is dependent in all transfers and all self-care. He is very embarrassed to be assisted with toileting, bathing, dressing, shaving, brushing his teeth, and even eating, by the young female nurses on the unit.

George lives in a single level home with his three younger brothers and his parents and grandmother. His mother is a homemaker and his father is a bus driver for the school system. The family is very close knit. Because George was injured in a school accident, the school's insurance will pay for all his medical care. What will you do to help George?

In order to use a client-centered approach, select one person in your group to "be" George. This person can then tell you about his roles, tasks, activities, interests, and priorities to assist you in developing your treatment plan and selecting appropriate therapeutic activities.

Table 17-1

MANUAL MUSCLE TEST

Muscle Action	Prime Movers	Spinal Cord Level	Strength in Left UE	Strength in Right UE
Scapula				
Abduction and upward rotation	serratus anterior	C5/C7	4	4
Abduction and downward rotation	middle trapezius	C2/C5	3	3
	rhomboids	C5	3	3
Elevation	levator scapulae	C3/C4	3	3
	upper trapezius	C2/C4		
Depression	lower trapezius	C2/C4	2	2
Shoulder	anterior deltoid	C5/C6	2	2
Flexion to 90 degrees	coracobrachialis	C6/C7	2	2
Extension/ hyperextension	latissimus dorsi	C5/C6	2	2
	teres major	C5/C6		
	posterior deltoid	C5/C6		
Abduction to 90 degrees	middle deltoid	C5/C6	2+	2
	supraspinatus	C5/C6	2+	2-
Adduction	pectoralis major	C5/T1	2+	1+
	latissimus dorsi	C6/C8		
Horizontal abduction	posterior deltoid	C5/C6	3-	2
Horizontal adduction	pectoralis major	C5/T1	2+	2
	anterior deltoid	C5/C6	2+	1+
	teres major	C5/C6		
Internal rotation	subscapularis	C5/C6	2	2
	pectoralis major	C5/T1		
	latissimus dorsi	C6/C8		
	teres major	C5/C6		
External rotation	infraspinatus	C5/C6	3-	2
	teres minor	C5	3-	2
Elbow	biceps	C5/C6	3-	2
Flexion with supination	brachialis	C5/C6		
Flexion/ forearm in neutral	brachioradialis	C5/C6	3+	1+
Extension	triceps	C6/C8	0	0
Forearm		C5/C6	2+	2-
Supination	biceps	C5/C7	2+	2-
	supinator			
Pronation	pronators teres	C6/C7	2+	1
	pronator quadratus	C7/T1	2+	1

Table 17-1 continued

Muscle Action	Prime Movers	Spinal Cord Level	Strength in Left UE	Strength in Right UE
Wrist	flexor carpi radialis	C6	0	0
Flexion	flexor carpi ulnaris	C8/T1		
Extension	extensor carpi radialis longus and brevis	C6/C7	2	0
	extensor carpi ulnaris	C7		

TUTORIAL SESSION SHEET

Case Study (Pt. Name, Dx.): George; C5/C6 Tetraplegia

Group Members' Names:

Facts/Knowledge	Learning Issues	Actions/Steps to Learn
What do you already know that will help you to approach this case?	What questions do you need to ask to learn about:	What are the plans to find the answers to your questions?
1. Individual client—roles, tasks, activities	1. Individual client—roles, tasks, activities	
2. The client's physical/sociocultural environment	2. The client's physical/sociocultural environment	
3. Clinical signs and symptoms, treatment for diagnosis	3. Clinical signs and symptoms, treatment for diagnosis	

Case Study Treatment Plan Sheet

Page 1

Case Study (Client Name; Dx.): *George; C5/C6 Tetraplegia*

Group Members' Names: _____

Deficits	Stage-Specific Cause	Short-Term Goals	Relates to which deficit	Functional Outcomes	Relates to which STG

Case Study Treatment Plan Sheet

Page 2

Case Study (Client Name; Dx.): *George; C5/C6 Tetraplegia*

Group Members' Names: _____

Short-Term Goals	Methods	Rationale	Tx Approach/ Frame of Reference	Specific Activity/ Modality

18

Niles

Retired Bank Teller with Posterior Cord Syndrome

Niles is a very independent gentleman 66 years of age. He is a retired banker. His wife passed away over a year ago. He lives alone in a second floor condominium (with no elevator) and does all his own housekeeping tasks. A few weeks prior to his surgery, he walked a mile around the condo every morning for exercise. He also swam leisurely almost every day. He enjoys coin collecting and loves to work with his computer and participate in chat rooms with people from all over the country. He also likes to manage his portfolio on the Internet.

Niles had surgery to remove a tumor on the posterior aspect of his spinal cord level C5 to C8. This has resulted in a posterior cord syndrome. The physician states the prognosis for recovery poor.

Niles has poor fine motor control in his hands secondary to sensory deficits. He requires moderate assistance with grooming, dressing, and bathing. He is dependent in homemaking tasks. Niles has a great deal of difficulty manipulating, picking up, and holding objects due to the poor fine motor control and sensory deficits. He also has difficulty opening, locking, and unlocking doors, and opening and closing closet doors, cabinets, and drawers. Presently, he is not participating in his hobbies of coin collecting and using the com-puter to access Internet chat rooms and manage his portfolio.

His daughter, Fay, lives three doors down in the same condominium complex. She is very supportive of him and very concerned about his ability to care for himself.

What will you do to help Niles?

In order to use a client-centered approach, select one person in your group to "be" Niles. This person can then tell you about his roles, tasks, activities, interests, and priorities to assist you in developing your treatment plan and selecting appropriate therapeutic activities.

TUTORIAL SESSION SHEET

Case Study (Pt. Name, Dx.): Niles; Posterior Cord Syndrome

Group Members' Names: _____

Facts/Knowledge

What do you already know that will help you to approach this case?

1. Individual client—roles, tasks, activities
2. The client's physical/sociocultural environment
3. Clinical signs and symptoms, treatment for diagnosis

Learning Issues

What questions do you need to ask to learn about:

1. Individual client—roles, tasks, activities
2. The client's physical/sociocultural environment
3. Clinical signs and symptoms, treatment for diagnosis

Actions/Steps to Learn

What are the plans to find the answers to your questions?

CASE STUDY TREATMENT PLAN SHEET

Case Study (Client Name; Dx.): Niles; Posterior Cord Syndrome

Group Members' Names: _____

Page 1

Deficits	Stage-Specific Cause	Short-Term Goals	Relates to which deficit	Functional Outcomes	Relates to which STG

CASE STUDY TREATMENT PLAN SHEET

Case Study (Client Name; Dx.): Niles; Posterior Cord Syndrome

Group Members' Names: _____

Short-Term Goals	Methods	Rationale	Tx Approach/ Frame of Reference	Specific Activity/ Modality

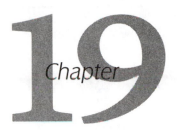

Chapter

19

Jim

Physical Education Instructor with T12 Paraplegia

Jim is a 22-year-old male who sustained a complete T12 paraplegia in an automobile accident. Prior to his injury, Jim just graduated from college and was working as a high school physical education instructor. He is single and lives alone at the present time. He has always been very independent and a risk taker. His hobbies include sports, particularly basketball, tennis, gymnastics, and sailing.

He and his fianceé were planning to get married in seven months. His fianceé, who is a high school math instructor, is very nervous about Jim's present condition and limitations. She is concerned about how their life plans have been interrupted. These plans included fixing up Jim's house, traveling during summer vacations, and eventually having children. She states they both have college loans to pay off and don't have much money saved as they have just entered the workforce.

Jim was transferred to your rehabilitation facility. He is medically stable. In reviewing the medical records you note that strength in all innervated musculature is in good range. Sensory deficits follow the classical pattern for his level of spinal injury. He has not yet achieved maximum functional level for his level of spinal injury. He will be in your rehabilitation facility for about 1 month.

He is particularly interested in being as independent as possible so he can manage his home and return to work, including being able to drive himself there. His home is a single level house in a rural area. He describes the home as old and small, with narrow doorways and door sills throughout. There are three steps to get in the front door and two steps to get in the house through the back door.

What will you do to help Jim?

In order to use a client-centered approach, select one person in your group to "be" Jim. This person can then tell you about his roles, tasks, activities, interests, and priorities to assist you in developing your treatment plan and selecting appropriate therapeutic activities.

TUTORIAL SESSION SHEET

Case Study (Pt. Name, Dx.): Jim; T12 Paraplegia

Group Members' Names: _____

Facts/Knowledge

What do you already know that will help you to approach this case?

1. Individual client—roles, tasks, activities
2. The client's physical/sociocultural environment
3. Clinical signs and symptoms, treatment for diagnosis

Learning Issues

What questions do you need to ask to learn about:

1. Individual client—roles, tasks, activities
2. The client's physical/sociocultural environment
3. Clinical signs and symptoms, treatment for diagnosis

Actions/Steps to Learn

What are the plans to find the answers to your questions?

CASE STUDY TREATMENT PLAN SHEET

Page 1

Case Study (Client Name; Dx.): Jim; T12 Paraplegia

Group Members' Names: _____

Deficits	Stage-Specific Cause	Short-Term Goals	Relates to which deficit	Functional Outcomes	Relates to which STG

CASE STUDY TREATMENT PLAN SHEET

Page 2

Case Study (Client Name; Dx.): Jim; T12 Paraplegia

Group Members' Names: _____

Short-Term Goals	Methods	Rationale	Tx Approach/ Frame of Reference	Specific Activity/ Modality

CASE STUDY TREATMENT PLAN SHEET

Case Study (Client Name; Dx.): Bob; Laceration of Extensor Tendons

Group Members' Names: _____

Short-Term Goals	Methods	Rationale	Tx Approach/ Frame of Reference	Specific Activity/ Modality

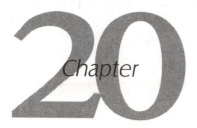

Chapter

Bob

TV Show Host with Laceration of Extensor Tendons

You own your own hand rehabilitation clinic. You receive referrals from several area physicians. The following prescription is faxed to you:

Name: Bob   Age: 47

Diagnosis: Extensor Tendon Injury

Orders: OT Evaluate and Treat

The next day, Bob comes for his first appointment. He has a bulky dressing on his right arm with another prescription from the physician that requests you remove the bulky dressing and fabricate a splint for Bob.

Bob tells you the following:

1. Bob is the host of a weekly home renovation and repair TV show.

2. Bob badly cut the back of his index finger and his middle finger while filming a segment on ceiling installation. He caught his fingers on an exposed nail 2 days ago. He had surgery to repair the severed tendon that same day.

3. Bob lives with his wife who is an executive producer of a cooking show. She works long hours and he rarely sees her. They have no children.

4. Bob will be expected to go to work every day but he isn't involved in the heavy construction aspect of the show. He is involved in the writing of each show and other administrative aspects.

5. Bob's job does involve a lot of politicking with network executives, particularly during Saturday fishing excursions on his boat. He needs to continue with these activities.

6. To relax, Bob loves to read.

7. You remove the bandage from Bob's hand and notice a 1/2 to 3/4 inch wound on the dorsal aspect of the 2nd and 3rd digits just distal to the MP joints. There are stitches in place.

You will treat Bob throughout the course of his recovery. What will you do to help Bob?

In order to use a client-centered approach, select one person in your group to "be" Bob. This person can then tell you about his roles, tasks, activities, interests, and priorities to assist you in developing your treatment plan and selecting appropriate therapeutic activities.

Occupational therapy s/p tendon repair generally follows a specific protocol. Identify the protocol you have chosen and indicate on your treatment plan approximate time frames, treatment methods, and activities for each stage of the protocol.

Tutorial Session Sheet

Case Study (Pt. Name, Dx.): Bob; Laceration of Extensor Tendons

Group Members' Names:

Facts/Knowledge	Learning Issues	Actions/Steps to Learn
What do you already know that will help you to approach this case? 1. Individual client—roles, tasks, activities 2. The client's physical/sociocultural environment 3. Clinical signs and symptoms, treatment for diagnosis	What questions do you need to ask to learn about: 1. Individual client—roles, tasks, activities 2. The client's physical/sociocultural environment 3. Clinical signs and symptoms, treatment for diagnosis	What are the plans to find the answers to your questions?

Case Study Treatment Plan Sheet

Page 1

Case Study (Client Name; Dx.): Bob; Laceration of Extensor Tendons

Group Members' Names: _____

Deficits	Stage Specific Cause	Short-Term Goals	Relates to which deficit	Functional Outcomes	Relates to which STG

21

Chapter

Mike

Architect with Laceration of Flexor Tendon

Case study developed by Karen Berry Ayala, MS, OTR/L

Mike is a 42-year-old architect referred to outpatient OT on May 19th s/p zone 2 flexor digitorum superficialis tendon laceration to the right middle finger. Mike injured his hand on May 18th and had surgery the same day.

Mike is right hand dominant. He was in good health prior to the accident. He lives at home with his wife, his six children, and his housekeeper. Mike's job responsibilities include drawing and designing blueprints, consulting with contractors and construction companies, and using a computer. In his spare time, Mike coaches his sons' football team, does all of the yard work, and leads camping trips for the local boy scout troop.

You will treat Mike throughout the course of his recovery. What will you do to help Mike?

In order to use a client-centered approach, select one person in your group to "be" Mike. This person can then tell you about his roles, tasks, activities, interests, and priorities to assist you in developing your treatment plan and selecting appropriate therapeutic activities.

Occupational therapy s/p tendon repair generally follows a specific protocol. Identify the protocol you have chosen and indicate on your treatment plan approximate time frames, treatment methods, and activities for each stage of the protocol.

TUTORIAL SESSION SHEET

Case Study (Pt. Name, Dx.): Mike; Laceration of Flexor Tendon

Group Members' Names: _____

Facts/Knowledge

What do you already know that will help you to approach this case?

1. Individual client—roles, tasks, activities
2. The client's physical/sociocultural environment
3. Clinical signs and symptoms, treatment for diagnosis

Learning Issues

What questions do you need to ask to learn about:

1. Individual client—roles, tasks, activities
2. The client's physical/sociocultural environment
3. Clinical signs and symptoms, treatment for diagnosis

Actions/Steps to Learn

What are the plans to find the answers to your questions?

CASE STUDY TREATMENT PLAN SHEET

Page 1

Case Study (Client Name; Dx.): Mike; Laceration of Flexor Tendon

Group Members' Names: _____

Deficits	Stage-Specific Cause	Short-Term Goals	Relates to which deficit	Functional Outcomes	Relates to which STG

CASE STUDY TREATMENT PLAN SHEET

Case Study (Client Name; Dx.): Mike; Laceration of Flexor Tension

Group Members' Names: _____

Short-Term Goals	Methods	Rationale	Tx Approach/ Frame of Reference	Specific Activity/ Modality

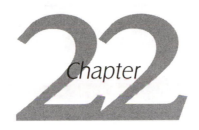

Chapter

Mick

Musician with a Fractured Humerus and an Ulnar Nerve Injury

Mick is a 35-year-old drummer in a rock and roll band. He is right hand dominant. On October 31st, he was involved in a stage accident while performing at the Fillmore East. One of the huge speakers fell on him, knocking him off the stage to the ground 6 feet below. The speaker then fell on top of him, fracturing his humerus and pinning his wrist to the ground, causing a crushing of the ulnar nerve (neurapraxia). He was taken to the emergency room. There the physician gave him a sling and swathe to immobilize his shoulder and a soft cast for his right wrist and hand and ordered OT to evaluate and treat. He arrives at your outpatient clinic on November 3rd.

During the evaluation, Mick is very preoccupied, answering his cell phone three times in a half hour to talk to his lawyer about the accident. He is concerned about his limitations in caring for himself and his inability to work in the band. Presently, the band is playing locally, but will go out on tour again in 2 weeks. He states that his wife has been supportive. She helps him with his daily living tasks. In spite of this, their relationship is becoming strained because of his anger and bitterness toward the stage hands who set up the equipment improperly.

Mick is complaining of severe pain (8 on a scale of 1 to 10) in his RUE. The right hand and wrist are moderately to severely edematous. You call the physician and he will allow you to start Codman's exercises for the shoulder and therapeutic exercises for the hand.

Mick has the following AROM limitations in the RUE: Measurement of shoulder motions was deferred. Mick lacks 30 degrees of active extension in the right elbow. He has 0 to 40 degrees of AROM in right wrist flexion and 0 to 35 degrees of AROM in wrist extension. Pronation measures 0 to 75 degrees of AROM and supination 0 to 40 degrees of AROM. AROM in

the right thumb flexion and extension is WFL. AROM of finger extension was WFL. The following AROM deficits were noted in finger flexion: 2nd and 3rd digits—MP joint 0 to 90; IP joint 0 to 95; DIP joint 0 to 60 degrees; 4th digit—MP joint 0 to 80; IP joint 0 to 85; DIP joint 0 to 50; 5th digit—MP joint 0 to 70; IP joint 0 to 90; DIP 0 to 50. He has limited opposition.

Strength testing of the right shoulder, elbow, forearm, and wrist musculature were deferred. Grip strength (as measured by the dynamometer) was 15 pounds in the right hand and 120 pounds in the left hand. Lateral pinch strength measured 13 pounds in the left and 7 pounds in the right. Three point pinch measured 10 pounds in the left and 4 pounds in the right.

He complains of severe hypersensitivity on the ulnar border of the right hand. He has diminished protective sensation on the volar side of the 4th and 5th digits. Fine motor coordination in the right hand is poor.

Mick needs assistance to manage all clothes closures. He is unable to cut his own food and he feeds himself using his nondominant left hand. He is unable to manage food containers but he states that this is okay because now it is his wife's job to do those things. Mick says that sometimes he thinks it is good that he has this time off because he had intended to write some songs, work in his organic vegetable garden, and create some tie dyed T-shirts. He would also love to tie flies and go fishing but then the pain is just making him miserable.

What will you do to help Mick?

In order to use a client-centered approach, select one person in your group to "be" Mick. This person can then tell you about his roles, tasks, activities, interests, and priorities to assist you in developing your treatment plan and selecting appropriate therapeutic activities.

TUTORIAL SESSION SHEET

Case Study (Pt. Name, Dx.): Mick; Fractured Humerus and an Ulnar Nerve Injury

Group Members' Names: _____

Facts/Knowledge

What do you already know that will help you to approach this case?

1. Individual client—roles, tasks, activities
2. The client's physical/sociocultural environment
3. Clinical signs and symptoms, treatment for diagnosis

Learning Issues

What questions do you need to ask to learn about:

1. Individual client—roles, tasks, activities
2. The client's physical/sociocultural environment
3. Clinical signs and symptoms, treatment for diagnosis

Actions/Steps to Learn

What are the plans to find the answers to your questions?

CASE STUDY TREATMENT PLAN SHEET

Page 1

Case Study (Client Name; Dx.): Mick; Fractured Humerus and an Ulnar Nerve Injury

Group Members' Names: _____

Deficits	Stage-Specific Cause	Short-Term Goals	Relates to which deficit	Functional Outcomes	Relates to which STG

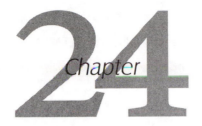

Chapter

Henry

Postal Service Worker with Complex Regional Pain Syndrome

Case study developed by Cheryl Acheson Reed, MS, OTR/L, CHT

Henry is a 53-year-old male who arrives at your clinic 10 minutes late for his initial appointment. He comes with a referring diagnosis of complex regional pain syndrome secondary to a healed ulnar head fracture of the RUE. The physician has ordered OT to evaluate and treat. His posture upon arriving is that of someone in a great deal of pain, extremely apprehensive, and splinting his RUE protectively across his chest. When you extend your hand to introduce yourself, he responds by offering his left hand and making a feeble verbal greeting. You ask him typical historical questions about how the injury happened, when it occurred, and the medical intervention he received. He responds angrily, stating that the medical establishment has been negligent; otherwise, he feels he should have recovered fully at this point. After all, the injury occurred 3 months ago and he does not feel that he should still be suffering residual effects. He relays that he has never been sick a day in his life. Upon further inquiry, you learn that he has never been seen in therapy. His physician had given him a written home exercise program but he forgot how to perform the exercises and misplaced the program. He just does not understand what has happened to his hand. Henry is upset because now he is incapable of feeding himself with his right hand in a normal fashion. He is only able to hold an eating utensil through the use of a gross grasp and is unable to hold a fork and knife adequately enough to cut food. Henry reports that he is unable to dress himself independently. His wife Trudy has to help him put his shirt and socks on and manage clothes fasteners on his shirt and pants. He has started wearing loafers because he cannot tie his shoes. He states that, due to the fact that he is right-handed, he has not been able to return to his position with UPS as he is unable to lift boxes for delivery and is unable to write the required reports.

During the interview, you explain what OT is and inform the client that he will be performing therapy gently and that he should not experience anything greater than mild discomfort. To place him further at ease, you inform him that he can request that you stop at any time and that you will comply. In essence, you place the client in control and reassure him. He responds by calming down somewhat.

As he begins to calm, he allows you to examine his hand. You note that his hand is edematous, with thin, shiny skin, and there are ridges in his nails. In addition, his palm exhibits hyperhidrosis.

As you progress further in the evaluation, you note that he appears to be hypersensitive on part of the ventral aspect of the hand. You evaluate him with the Semmes-Weinstein and determine that he has diminished protective sensation on the distal tops of the ring and small fingers of the hand.

Upon observing the resting posture of his hands, you note a normal left hand. However, resting position of the right hand indicates there is some hyperextension of the fourth and fifth metacarpophalangeal joints, with flexion of the IP joints of fourth and fifth digits. You passively place the MP joints of the client's ring and small fingers into flexion and request that he extend his digits. At this point, the client is able to adequately extend the interphalangeal joints. Upon being asked to extend the fourth and fifth digits with no external support, the client merely increases the clawlike posture. Henry also has a positive Froment's sign. You then examine the joints passively. In doing so, you find that AROM of the shoulder is WNL. However, the forearm is severely limited in supination at 40 degrees. Pronation is WNL, as is elbow flexion and extension. AROM of the wrist is limited in all planes, including flexion (35 degrees), extension (40 degrees), ulnar

Table 24-1
AROM MEASUREMENTS

	Thumb	Index	Long	Ring	Small
MP	0 to 35	0 to 80	0 to 75	10 to 62	15 to 60
PIP	0 to 25	0 to 95	-10 to 92	-24 to 60	-15 to 52
DIP		0 to 58	0 to 60	0 to 42	0 to 54
TPM	60	233	217	150	166

Table 24-2
PINCH STRENGTH MEASURES

	Lateral	3 Jaw Chuck	Tip Pinch
Left	13 pounds	8 pounds	6 pounds
Right	5 pounds	3 pounds	2 pounds

deviation (12 degrees), and radial deviation (5 degrees) (Table 24-1). The digits are also limited.

No significant differences in active ROM were noted when stabilization was provided, with some exceptions (support of 4th and 5th MP joints in flexion yields full IP extension). Abduction and adduction of the digits is limited and the client has difficulty assuming an intrinsic plus position. PROM was not tested at this time due to Henry's apprehension and attempts to avoid pain and build trust.

Definitive manual muscle testing is deferred due to the client's limited ROM. Strength testing of the hand is administered, though, with three trials of each hand with the dynamometer. You are careful to insure that the client assumes the proper posture during testing.

Results of the right hand are:
- 1st trial—17 pounds
- 2nd trial—15 pounds
- 3rd trial—15 pounds

Results of the left hand are:
- 1st trial—55 pounds
- 2nd trial—52 pounds
- 3rd trial—53 pounds

Pinch strength measures are found in Table 24-2.

To test edema, you use the volumeter, again being certain to have the client assume the correct posture. There is a water displacement recording of 740ml on the right and 675ml on the left.

In determining the pain that Henry is experiencing, you use the McGill Pain Questionnaire. The client indicates he has a significant amount of pain. No deficit is noted when you perform the Allen test.

The client states his priority is to be able to care for his personal needs. What will you do to help Henry?

In order to use a client-centered approach, select one person in your group to "be" Henry. This person can then tell you about his roles, tasks, activities, interests, and priorities to assist you in developing your treatment plan and selecting appropriate therapeutic activities.

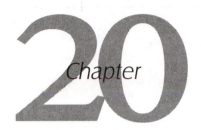

Bob

TV Show Host with Laceration of Extensor Tendons

You own your own hand rehabilitation clinic. You receive referrals from several area physicians. The following prescription is faxed to you:

Name: Bob   Age: 47
Diagnosis: Extensor Tendon Injury
Orders: OT Evaluate and Treat

The next day, Bob comes for his first appointment. He has a bulky dressing on his right arm with another prescription from the physician that requests you remove the bulky dressing and fabricate a splint for Bob.

Bob tells you the following:

1. Bob is the host of a weekly home renovation and repair TV show.

2. Bob badly cut the back of his index finger and his middle finger while filming a segment on ceiling installation. He caught his fingers on an exposed nail 2 days ago. He had surgery to repair the severed tendon that same day.

3. Bob lives with his wife who is an executive producer of a cooking show. She works long hours and he rarely sees her. They have no children.

4. Bob will be expected to go to work every day but he isn't involved in the heavy construction aspect of the show. He is involved in the writing of each show and other administrative aspects.

5. Bob's job does involve a lot of politicking with network executives, particularly during Saturday fishing excursions on his boat. He needs to continue with these activities.

6. To relax, Bob loves to read.

7. You remove the bandage from Bob's hand and notice a 1/2 to 3/4 inch wound on the dorsal aspect of the 2nd and 3rd digits just distal to the MP joints. There are stitches in place.

You will treat Bob throughout the course of his recovery. What will you do to help Bob?

In order to use a client-centered approach, select one person in your group to "be" Bob. This person can then tell you about his roles, tasks, activities, interests, and priorities to assist you in developing your treatment plan and selecting appropriate therapeutic activities.

Occupational therapy s/p tendon repair generally follows a specific protocol. Identify the protocol you have chosen and indicate on your treatment plan approximate time frames, treatment methods, and activities for each stage of the protocol.

TUTORIAL SESSION SHEET

Case Study (Pt. Name, Dx.): Bob; Laceration of Extensor Tendons

Group Members' Names: _____

Facts/Knowledge	Learning Issues	Actions/Steps to Learn
What do you already know that will help you to approach this case? 1. Individual client—roles, tasks, activities 2. The client's physical/sociocultural environment 3. Clinical signs and symptoms, treatment for diagnosis	What questions do you need to ask to learn about: 1. Individual client—roles, tasks, activities 2. The client's physical/sociocultural environment 3. Clinical signs and symptoms, treatment for diagnosis	What are the plans to find the answers to your questions?

21 Chapter

Mike

Architect with Laceration of Flexor Tendon

Case study developed by Karen Berry Ayala, MS, OTR/L

Mike is a 42-year-old architect referred to outpatient OT on May 19th s/p zone 2 flexor digitorum superficialis tendon laceration to the right middle finger. Mike injured his hand on May 18th and had surgery the same day.

Mike is right hand dominant. He was in good health prior to the accident. He lives at home with his wife, his six children, and his housekeeper. Mike's job responsibilities include drawing and designing blueprints, consulting with contractors and construction companies, and using a computer. In his spare time, Mike coaches his sons' football team, does all of the yard work, and leads camping trips for the local boy scout troop.

You will treat Mike throughout the course of his recovery. What will you do to help Mike?

In order to use a client-centered approach, select one person in your group to "be" Mike. This person can then tell you about his roles, tasks, activities, interests, and priorities to assist you in developing your treatment plan and selecting appropriate therapeutic activities.

Occupational therapy s/p tendon repair generally follows a specific protocol. Identify the protocol you have chosen and indicate on your treatment plan approximate time frames, treatment methods, and activities for each stage of the protocol.

TUTORIAL SESSION SHEET

Case Study (Pt. Name, Dx.): *Mike; Laceration of Flexor Tendon*

Group Members' Names: _____

Facts/Knowledge	Learning Issues	Actions/Steps to Learn
What do you already know that will help you to approach this case? 1. Individual client—roles, tasks, activities 2. The client's physical/sociocultural environment 3. Clinical signs and symptoms, treatment for diagnosis	What questions do you need to ask to learn about: 1. Individual client—roles, tasks, activities 2. The client's physical/sociocultural environment 3. Clinical signs and symptoms, treatment for diagnosis	What are the plans to find the answers to your questions?

CASE STUDY TREATMENT PLAN SHEET

Page 1

Case Study (Client Name; Dx.): Mike; Laceration of Flexor Tendon

Group Members' Names: _____

Deficits	Stage-Specific Cause	Short-Term Goals	Relates to which deficit	Functional Outcomes	Relates to which STG

Case Study Treatment Plan Sheet

Case Study (Client Name; Dx.): Mike; Laceration of Flexor Tension

Group Members' Names: _____

Short-Term Goals	Methods	Rationale	Tx Approach/ Frame of Reference	Specific Activity/ Modality

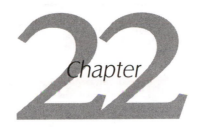

Mick

Musician with a Fractured Humerus and an Ulnar Nerve Injury

Mick is a 35-year-old drummer in a rock and roll band. He is right hand dominant. On October 31st, he was involved in a stage accident while performing at the Fillmore East. One of the huge speakers fell on him, knocking him off the stage to the ground 6 feet below. The speaker then fell on top of him, fracturing his humerus and pinning his wrist to the ground, causing a crushing of the ulnar nerve (neurapraxia). He was taken to the emergency room. There the physician gave him a sling and swathe to immobilize his shoulder and a soft cast for his right wrist and hand and ordered OT to evaluate and treat. He arrives at your outpatient clinic on November 3rd.

During the evaluation, Mick is very preoccupied, answering his cell phone three times in a half hour to talk to his lawyer about the accident. He is concerned about his limitations in caring for himself and his inability to work in the band. Presently, the band is playing locally, but will go out on tour again in 2 weeks. He states that his wife has been supportive. She helps him with his daily living tasks. In spite of this, their relationship is becoming strained because of his anger and bitterness toward the stage hands who set up the equipment improperly.

Mick is complaining of severe pain (8 on a scale of 1 to 10) in his RUE. The right hand and wrist are moderately to severely edematous. You call the physician and he will allow you to start Codman's exercises for the shoulder and therapeutic exercises for the hand.

Mick has the following AROM limitations in the RUE: Measurement of shoulder motions was deferred. Mick lacks 30 degrees of active extension in the right elbow. He has 0 to 40 degrees of AROM in right wrist flexion and 0 to 35 degrees of AROM in wrist extension. Pronation measures 0 to 75 degrees of AROM and supination 0 to 40 degrees of AROM. AROM in

the right thumb flexion and extension is WFL. AROM of finger extension was WFL. The following AROM deficits were noted in finger flexion: 2nd and 3rd digits—MP joint 0 to 90; IP joint 0 to 95; DIP joint 0 to 60 degrees; 4th digit—MP joint 0 to 80; IP joint 0 to 85; DIP joint 0 to 50; 5th digit—MP joint 0 to 70; IP joint 0 to 90; DIP 0 to 50. He has limited opposition.

Strength testing of the right shoulder, elbow, forearm, and wrist musculature were deferred. Grip strength (as measured by the dynamometer) was 15 pounds in the right hand and 120 pounds in the left hand. Lateral pinch strength measured 13 pounds in the left and 7 pounds in the right. Three point pinch measured 10 pounds in the left and 4 pounds in the right.

He complains of severe hypersensitivity on the ulnar border of the right hand. He has diminished protective sensation on the volar side of the 4th and 5th digits. Fine motor coordination in the right hand is poor.

Mick needs assistance to manage all clothes closures. He is unable to cut his own food and he feeds himself using his nondominant left hand. He is unable to manage food containers but he states that this is okay because now it is his wife's job to do those things. Mick says that sometimes he thinks it is good that he has this time off because he had intended to write some songs, work in his organic vegetable garden, and create some tie dyed T-shirts. He would also love to tie flies and go fishing but then the pain is just making him miserable.

What will you do to help Mick?

In order to use a client-centered approach, select one person in your group to "be" Mick. This person can then tell you about his roles, tasks, activities, interests, and priorities to assist you in developing your treatment plan and selecting appropriate therapeutic activities.

TUTORIAL SESSION SHEET

Case Study (Pt. Name, Dx.): Mick; Fractured Humerus and an Ulnar Nerve Injury

Group Members' Names: _____

Facts/Knowledge

What do you already know that will help you to approach this case?

1. Individual client—roles, tasks, activities
2. The client's physical/sociocultural environment
3. Clinical signs and symptoms, treatment for diagnosis

Learning Issues

What questions do you need to ask to learn about:

1. Individual client—roles, tasks, activities
2. The client's physical/sociocultural environment
3. Clinical signs and symptoms, treatment for diagnosis

Actions/Steps to Learn

What are the plans to find the answers to your questions?

CASE STUDY TREATMENT PLAN SHEET

Page 1

Case Study (Client Name; Dx.): *Mick; Fractured Humerus and an Ulnar Nerve Injury*

Group Members' Names: _____

Deficits	Stage-Specific Cause	Short-Term Goals	Relates to which deficit	Functional Outcomes	Relates to which STG

CASE STUDY TREATMENT PLAN SHEET

Page 2

Case Study (Client Name; Dx.): Mick; Fractured Humerus and an Ulnar Nerve Injury

Group Members' Names: _____

Short-Term Goals	Methods	Rationale	Tx Approach/ Frame of Reference	Specific Activity/ Modality

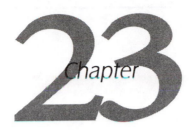

Ray

Retiree with a Radial Nerve Injury

Ray underwent routine surgery under general anesthesia. When he awoke from surgery, he noticed that his right hand was "floppy" and that he was unable to extend his right wrist or fingers. You note that he cannot supinate his forearm. A surgical nurse in the hospital mentioned that he was positioned on the surgery table with his right arm hanging off the table and maybe this had something to do with the problem. There was a red mark near the posterior and lateral aspect just above the elbow. He is left hand dominant.

Ray is a recent retiree who enjoys playing cards and going to the racetrack with his buddies. He lives with his wife of 3 years (second marriage for both). He and his wife are both very independent and private people. They do not spend a lot of time together.

What will you do to help Ray?

In order to use a client-centered approach, select one person in your group to "be" Ray. This person can then tell you about his roles, tasks, activities, interests, and priorities to assist you in developing your treatment plan and selecting appropriate therapeutic activities.

TUTORIAL SESSION SHEET

Case Study (Pt. Name, Dx.): Ray; Radial Nerve Injury

Group Members' Names: _____

Facts/Knowledge	Learning Issues	Actions/Steps to Learn
What do you already know that will help you to approach this case? 1. Individual client—roles, tasks, activities 2. The client's physical/sociocultural environment 3. Clinical signs and symptoms, treatment for diagnosis	What questions do you need to ask to learn about: 1. Individual client—roles, tasks, activities 2. The client's physical/sociocultural environment 3. Clinical signs and symptoms, treatment for diagnosis	What are the plans to find the answers to your questions?

CASE STUDY TREATMENT PLAN SHEET

Case Study (Client Name; Dx.): Ray; Radial Nerve Injury

Group Members' Names: _____

Page 1

Deficits	Stage-Specific Cause	Short-Term Goals	Relates to which deficit	Functional Outcomes	Relates to which STG

CASE STUDY TREATMENT PLAN SHEET

Page 2

Case Study (Client Name; Dx.): *Ray; Radial Nerve Injury*

Group Members' Names: _____

Short-Term Goals	Methods	Rationale	Tx Approach/ Frame of Reference	Specific Activity/ Modality

CASE STUDY TREATMENT PLAN SHEET

Page 2

Case Study (Client Name; Dx.): Bob; Laceration of Extensor Tendons

Group Members' Names: _____

Short-Term Goals	Methods	Rationale	Tx Approach/ Frame of Reference	Specific Activity/ Modality

CASE STUDY TREATMENT PLAN SHEET

Page 1

Case Study (Client Name; Dx.): Bob; Laceration of Extensor Tendons

Group Members' Names: _____

Deficits	Stage Specific Cause	Short-Term Goals	Relates to which deficit	Functional Outcomes	Relates to which STG

CASE STUDY TREATMENT PLAN SHEET

Page 1

Case Study (Client Name; Dx.): Dee; Repetitive Strain Injury

Group Members' Names: _____

Deficits	Stage-Specific Cause	Short-Term Goals	Relates to which deficit	Functional Outcomes	Relates to which STG

CASE STUDY TREATMENT PLAN SHEET

Case Study (Client Name; Dx.): Dee; Repetitive Strain Injury

Group Members' Names: _____

Short-Term Goals	Methods	Rationale	Tx Approach/ Frame of Reference	Specific Activity/ Modality

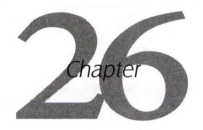

Chapter 26

Colby

Lab Employee at Risk

Case study developed by Karen Berry Ayala, MS, OTR/L

Colby is a 45-year-old man working in a research laboratory at a biotechnology corporation. Due to the Food and Drug Administration (FDA) regulations, the laboratory that Colby works in must be maintained at 62 degrees. The FDA mandates that Colby must keep his arms above his waist at all times due to risk of disrupting the carefully controlled air-flow. The FDA also mandates that all employees wear disposable lab coats, hair nets, shoe covers, and two pairs of latex gloves. Because Colby is handling sterile equipment, he must continuously clean his hands with rubbing alcohol. Colby works 10-hour shifts 4 days a week so that he can spend quality time with his wife and 3 daughters.

Recently, Colby has been complaining of numbness in all digits of both hands. His fingers appear slightly blue in color and feel cold to the touch. He has impaired fine and gross motor skills in both hands as well. He is very worried that he will not be able to continue to support his family if this problem continues.

Colby filed a worker's compensation claim and has been authorized for four OT visits. What can you do to help Colby?

In order to use a client-centered approach, select one person in your group to "be" Colby. This person can then tell you about his roles, tasks, activities, interests, and priorities to assist you in developing your treatment plan and selecting appropriate therapeutic activities.

TUTORIAL SESSION SHEET

Case Study (Pt. Name, Dx.): Colby; Lab Employee at Risk

Group Members' Names: _____

Facts/Knowledge	Learning Issues	Actions/Steps to Learn
What do you already know that will help you to approach this case?	What questions do you need to ask to learn about:	What are the plans to find the answers to your questions?
1. Individual client—roles, tasks, activities	1. Individual client—roles, tasks, activities	
2. The client's physical/sociocultural environment	2. The client's physical/sociocultural environment	
3. Clinical signs and symptoms, treatment for diagnosis	3. Clinical signs and symptoms, treatment for diagnosis	

CASE STUDY TREATMENT PLAN SHEET

Page 1

Case Study (Client Name; Dx.): *Colby; Lab Employee at Risk*

Group Members' Names: _____

Deficits	Stage-Specific Cause	Short-Term Goals	Relates to which deficit	Functional Outcomes	Relates to which STG

CASE STUDY TREATMENT PLAN SHEET

Case Study (Client Name; Dx.): Colby; Lab Employee at Risk

Group Members' Names: _____

Short-Term Goals	Methods	Rationale	Tx Approach/ Frame of Reference	Specific Activity/ Modality

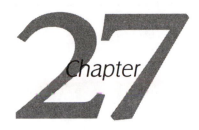

Chapter 27

Lynn

Fieldwork Coordinator with Carpal Tunnel Syndrome

Lynn works as a fieldwork coordinator in a local university. She is experiencing symptoms of paresthesia and pain which began in her index and long fingers of her right hand and later included her thumb and ring fingers. These symptoms are more prominent at night. She asks you if this problem has been caused by her working on the computer all day long. Lynn states that she requires frequent rest periods to allow the symptoms to subside before resuming job tasks. She has difficulty typing for longer than 30 to 40 minutes without experiencing tingling and pain in her left fingers. This has reduced her efficiency in performing her job. Lynn also complains of occasional neck pain and back pain. She notices that it is particularly difficult to get out of her chair to go home after working all day long. This has reduced her competency and efficiency in performing her job. She is also unable to lift the heavy boxes of computer paper and other nursing and office supplies. She wonders if something can be done to improve the set up of her office so that she won't have these problems.

Lynn has been married to her husband for 32 years. They have two grown children. They both live close by. Lynn enjoys gardening, embroidery and other needlework, and watching TV. She is the primary homemaker. Lynn complains that she has a lot of pain in her hands when cooking and has had increasing difficulty cutting food and opening food containers. She also states that she has difficulty carrying heavy objects with both her hands such as groceries and lifting her grandchildren. Her husband has been very helpful the past few weeks, assisting with the cooking and cleaning chores, however, she feels this is wearing thin. Lynn is very anxious. She needs someone to help her. What will you do to help Lynn?

In order to use a client-centered approach, select one person in your group to "be" Lynn. This person can then tell you about her roles, tasks, activities, interests, and priorities to assist you in developing your treatment plan and selecting appropriate therapeutic activities.

TUTORIAL SESSION SHEET

Case Study (Pt. Name, Dx.): Lynn; Carpal Tunnel Syndrome

Group Members' Names: _____

Facts/Knowledge

What do you already know that will help you to approach this case?

1. Individual client—roles, tasks, activities
2. The client's physical/sociocultural environment
3. Clinical signs and symptoms, treatment for diagnosis

Learning Issues

What questions do you need to ask to learn about:

1. Individual client—roles, tasks, activities
2. The client's physical/sociocultural environment
3. Clinical signs and symptoms, treatment for diagnosis

Actions/Steps to Learn

What are the plans to find the answers to your questions?

CASE STUDY TREATMENT PLAN SHEET

Case Study (Client Name; Dx.): Lynn; Carpal Tunnel Syndrome

Group Members' Names: _____

Page 1

Deficits	Stage-Specific Cause	Short-Term Goals	Relates to which deficit	Functional Outcomes	Relates to which STG

CASE STUDY TREATMENT PLAN SHEET

Case Study (Client Name; Dx.): Lynn; Carpal Tunnel Syndrome

Group Members' Names: _____

Short-Term Goals	Methods	Rationale	Tx Approach/ Frame of Reference	Specific Activity/ Modality

28
Chapter

Grant

Food Service Worker with Multiple Sclerosis

Case study developed by Barbara L. Kornblau, JD, OTR/L, FAOTA, DAAPM, ABDA, CDMS, CCM

Grant is 35 years old and was recently diagnosed with multiple sclerosis (MS). Grant was recently hospitalized for 1 week where the diagnosis of MS was made.

He works as a prep cook in the kitchen of a large resort hotel on the grounds of the Fun 'N Sun Resort. He has worked for the company for 7 years and has been a well-liked employee, winning employee of the month 12 times. Leading up to the diagnosis of MS were a series of falls and a problem with balance. Grant now uses a cane and is a little more stable. The Chef, the boss of the kitchen, has been concerned that Grant's problems were due to drinking.

Grant's doctor has told him he can return to work. His doctor gives him a note to give to the Chef as follows:

"Grant is able to return to his job with the following work restrictions: no work around steam and heat, no prolonged standing, no more than 40 hours of work per week, no lifting over 20 pounds. Client fatigues easily."

Grant isn't sure if he can do his job with the restrictions but is very motivated to return to his job.

The Chef reads the note and panics. He likes Grant and wants to help him out but he is at a loss at what to do. He is still unaware of Grant's diagnosis. He feels the apparent drinking problem warrants dismissal rather than a lighter workload. The Chef contacts the human resources director and many hours are spent discussing the issue "Can Grant still do his job with these restrictions?" The job description written 20 years ago is of little help in making a decision. After some time, the human resources director's secretary, whose sister is an OT, suggests that the resort call an OT for assistance. They call you with the following questions:

1. What is Grant capable of doing?
2. Can Grant return to his position as a prep cook?
3. Will he need accommodations to do his job?
4. What are the hotel's obligations to Grant?

They hire you to consult, asking for a report in 1 week. What can you do to help the hotel understand and deal with this situation?

Develop a report describing what consultative services you have provided. In this report, answer the hotel's questions and provide them with information that management needs to be aware of when dealing with this situation.

TUTORIAL SESSION SHEET

Case Study (Pt. Name, Dx.): Grant; Worker with Multiple Sclerosis

Group Members' Names: _____

Facts/Knowledge

What do you already know that will help you to approach this case?

1. Individual client—roles, tasks, activities
2. The client's physical/sociocultural environment
3. Clinical signs and symptoms, treatment for diagnosis

Learning Issues

What questions do you need to ask to learn about:

1. Individual client—roles, tasks, activities
2. The client's physical/sociocultural environment
3. Clinical signs and symptoms, treatment for diagnosis

Actions/Steps to Learn

What are the plans to find the answers to your questions?

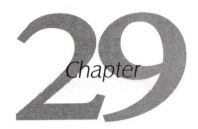

Moore Pharmaceuticals

Workers at Risk

Case study developed by Barbara L. Kornblau, JD, OTR/L, FAOTA, DAAPM, ABDA, CDMS, CCM

Moore Pharmaceuticals manufactures high tech surgical equipment. Over the past 5 years there has been a steady increase in on-the-job injuries among employees working in the prat division. For purposes of this case study, a prat (fictitious object) is made of metal and glass. A prat weighs 35 pounds, is cylindrical in shape, measures 2.5 feet in diameter, and 3 feet in length. The highest incidence has been in reported cases of back sprains and strains, various UE nerve entrapment syndromes, and some radiculopathies. The company has tried an education program as a way of preventing all of the injuries. This program consists of hanging posters everywhere in the plant describing and illustrating proper lifting techniques, but this has done nothing to curb the increasing incidence of reported injuries.

Because of the increase in reported injuries, worker's compensation claims have increased by 75% over the last 5 years, while the company's claim payouts have increased by over 100% in just the last 2 years. To make matters worse, recently a group of employees got together and filed a series of charges with the Equal Employment Opportunity Commission (EEOC). These employees claim the company refused to take them back to work following their injuries, because they had not made a 100% recovery to their pre-accident condition. In a panic, with the Occupational Safety and Health Administration (OSHA), EEOC,

and worker's compensation breathing down its neck, the company calls you.

You decide to visit the job site. You discover that many workers are assigned to the prat assembly line. The prats are hung on the assembly line located overhead. Several workers are required to add some parts to the core of the prat using power tools to tighten nuts and bolts. Then, other workers remove hanging prats from the line which is located overhead and place them on flats on another line, located at shoulder height, approximately 4 feet away from their work stations. At the end of the line, other workers take the prats off the flat and place them in packing boxes located on the floor. You remove a single prat, and place it on the flat, straining your shoulder. What will you do to help Moore Pharmaceuticals solve this problem?

Develop a comprehensive proposal to the company including the following:

1. What are the company's problems?
2. What steps would you take to solve the company's problems?
3. How will implementation of your suggestions benefit the company and its employees?
4. What suggestions might you have for the company for the future?

TUTORIAL SESSION SHEET

Case Study (Pt. Name, Dx.): Moore Pharmaceuticals; Workers at Risk

Group Members' Names: _____

Facts/Knowledge	Learning Issues	Actions/Steps to Learn
What do you already know that will help you to approach this case? 1. Individual client—roles, tasks, activities 2. The client's physical/sociocultural environment 3. Clinical signs and symptoms, treatment for diagnosis	What questions do you need to ask to learn about: 1. Individual client—roles, tasks, activities 2. The client's physical/sociocultural environment 3. Clinical signs and symptoms, treatment for diagnosis	What are the plans to find the answers to your questions?

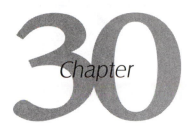

Chapter 30

Jack

Prison Guard with Severe Burns

Three days ago, Jack was helping to fill a propane tank at the local gas station when an explosion occurred. He loved to barbeque and was getting the tank filled for a block party where he was going to do the cooking for over 100 people. Jack was severely burned on the left side of his body in the explosion. As the fire flashed into his face, he covered his face with his hands. As a result, he received second and third degree burns on the dorsum of both hands. He also suffered second and third degree burns on the dorsal surface of both his forearms, the anterior side and left side of his neck, his left shoulder and axilla area, his chest and abdomen (primarily the left side), and the anterior portion of both legs. The burns covered 30% of his body.

You are the OT on the acute burn unit. The physician has ordered OT. The physician specifically requested appropriate splints and positioning devices to be fabricated. The physician also wants OT to maximize the client's functional ability.

Jack is 36 years old. He is married with two young children, one boy who is 4 years old and one girl who is 2 years old. Another child is on the way. Jack works as a prison guard in a medium security prison. He has a great deal of sick time available and can also "borrow" time from a "sick day pool" if he needs to.

Jack is a very loving husband and father. He especially adores his son and enjoys teaching him how to play catch. He has been a coach in a pee wee baseball league and is looking forward to the day his son can join the team. Jack's other love is his 1963 Corvette that he is restoring. He is in the process of restoring the interior and body.

Jack is anxious to return to work and to his leisure activities. What will you do to help Jack?

In order to use a client-centered approach, select one person in your group to "be" Jack. This person can then tell you about his roles, tasks, activities, interests, and priorities to assist you in developing your treatment plan and selecting appropriate therapeutic activities.

TUTORIAL SESSION SHEET

Case Study (Pt. Name, Dx.): Jack; Severe Burns

Group Members' Names: _____

Facts/Knowledge	Learning Issues	Actions/Steps to Learn
What do you already know that will help you to approach this case?	What questions do you need to ask to learn about:	What are the plans to find the answers to your questions?
1. Individual client—roles, tasks, activities	1. Individual client—roles, tasks, activities	
2. The client's physical/sociocultural environment	2. The client's physical/sociocultural environment	
3. Clinical signs and symptoms, treatment for diagnosis	3. Clinical signs and symptoms, treatment for diagnosis	

CASE STUDY TREATMENT PLAN SHEET

Page 1

Case Study (Client Name; Dx.): *Jack; Severe Burns*

Group Members' Names: _____

Deficits	Stage-Specific Cause	Short-Term Goals	Relates to which deficit	Functional Outcomes	Relates to which STG

CASE STUDY TREATMENT PLAN SHEET

Case Study (Client Name; Dx.): Jack; Severe Burns

Group Members' Names: _____

Short-Term Goals	Methods	Rationale	Tx Approach/ Frame of Reference	Specific Activity/ Modality

31

Lou

Airline Reservation Clerk with Multiple Sclerosis

On May 28th, Lou was referred to home health OT with a diagnosis of MS. Lou is 35 years old. He was diagnosed when he was 29 years old. Lou had an exacerbation and was discharged 2 days ago after a 2 week stay.

Lou, a bachelor, lives in a first floor apartment. His mother lives in the apartment across the hall. She is very supportive, does his shopping, cleaning, his laundry, and most of his cooking for him. As Lou no longer drives, she had been transporting him to work and other places.

Lou works as an airline reservation clerk for Flyaway Airlines. The company has been very supportive of Lou, giving him time off as he needs and allowing him to work at home when he is unable to get to work. Lou is anxious to get back to work because he likes to socialize with his coworkers.

Lou is cooperative, pleasant, and alert. He is oriented x 3, and long- and short-term memory are intact. Lou is very motivated to be independent, however he lacks safety awareness. Lou has diplopia. He likes to read mystery novels so this is very disturbing to him. It also interferes with his work; he uses the computer for work and has difficulty reading the screen.

Lou is right handed. His left hand is functional for ADL. He has ataxia in his RUE. He is able to use the RUE as an active stabilizer, but has difficulty using it for fine motor tasks such as writing. He has difficulty feeding himself with his right hand, spilling food frequently. He shaves himself with an electric razor, although with difficulty secondary to the ataxia.

Lou has a standard adult wheelchair. He propels this wheelchair around the apartment with his feet. Maneuvering the wheelchair around the apartment is difficult due to the plush carpeting on the floor and also the limited space. He is unable to get into the bathroom with the wheelchair because of the narrow width of the doorway. The walls are suffering with numerous dents and scuff marks. Lou has installed railings around his apartment so he can walk around supporting himself on the railings. Lou has a walker but does not like to use it.

Lou has fair plus dynamic sitting balance and fair to poor dynamic standing balance. He requires contact guard for safe transfers from the wheelchair to the bed and minimal assistance from the wheelchair to the car. He requires moderate assistance to transfer in and out of his shower stall. Lou prefers showering, but has limited endurance which affects his standing tolerance. He has safety bars in the shower which help support him as his mother bathes him. He would like to be able to bathe himself.

Lou is able to don a pullover shirt, but he requires moderate assistance to don pants secondary to limited dynamic sitting balance and inability to manage the zipper and button his pants. He also requires moderate assistance to don and doff socks and sneakers secondary to limited ability to maintain sitting balance when reaching to his feet.

Lou would like to be able to get a simple meal for himself. His mother works part-time and cannot always be there to fix his meals. Presently, his mother has to prepare all his meals and serve them. If she isn't there, he doesn't eat.

What will you do to help Lou?

In order to use a client-centered approach, select one person in your group to "be" Lou. This person can then tell you about his roles, tasks, activities, interests, and priorities to assist you in developing your treatment plan and selecting appropriate therapeutic activities.

TUTORIAL SESSION SHEET

Case Study (Pt. Name, Dx.): Lou; Multiple Sclerosis

Group Members' Names: _____

Facts/Knowledge

What do you already know that will help you to approach this case?

1. Individual client—roles, tasks, activities
2. The client's physical/sociocultural environment
3. Clinical signs and symptoms, treatment for diagnosis

Learning Issues

What questions do you need to ask to learn about:

1. Individual client—roles, tasks, activities
2. The client's physical/sociocultural environment
3. Clinical signs and symptoms, treatment for diagnosis

Actions/Steps to Learn

What are the plans to find the answers to your questions?

CASE STUDY TREATMENT PLAN SHEET

Page 1

Case Study (Client Name; Dx.): Lou; Multiple Sclerosis

Group Members' Names: _____

Deficits	Stage-Specific Cause	Short-Term Goals	Relates to which deficit	Functional Outcomes	Relates to which STG

CASE STUDY TREATMENT PLAN SHEET

Case Study (Client Name; Dx.): Lou; Multiple Sclerosis

Group Members' Names: _____

Short-Term Goals	Methods	Rationale	Tx Approach/ Frame of Reference	Specific Activity/ Modality

32

Thomas

Retired Postal Worker with Left Hemiplegia

Thomas is a 66-year-old male who was admitted to the hospital on May 21st after having suffered a cerebrovascular accident (CVA). On May 21st, Thomas developed weakness on his left side. His wife took him to the hospital where he was diagnosed with a CVA.

Thomas, a college graduate, recently retired from the U.S. Postal Service. He enjoys stamp collecting, golfing, playing cards with his buddies, and visiting the racetrack. Thomas' spouse is healthy and supportive. His wife has always done all the homemaking chores while he has always taken care of the yard work. He takes a great deal of pride in his tomato garden. He and his wife have talked about hiring help for the outside work, however, Thomas is very particular about the quality of the work and is reluctant to let someone else take care of his yard and garden. Thomas is very concerned that his friends will withdraw from him as they have done so in the past when one of the group has taken sick. He and his wife have one son who lives in the same town.

Thomas is alert, oriented to person but not to place or time. His short-term memory is mildly impaired and long-term memory is intact. He is impulsive and his safety awareness is poor. Thomas is able to express himself verbally. He is able to follow most commands and can attend for a full 30-minute therapy session with occasional redirection to the task.

Thomas has a left visual field cut and has difficulty tracking moving objects to the left of midline. He was unable to read a paragraph and complains of his "eyes jumping" when attempting to read his golfing magazine. He wears eyeglasses for reading. He is planning to make an appointment with his eye doctor to see if the prescription needs to be changed.

Thomas's functional status is as follows:

1. General endurance is fair.
2. Feeds himself when his food is cut with occasional reminders to look to the left side of his plate. He occasionally pockets food in the left side of his mouth.
3. Supervision to minimal assistance with grooming tasks. He needed assistance to find grooming aids in a cluttered drawer.
4. Moderate assistance with bathing tasks and with dressing, including locating parts of his clothing and securing fasteners.
5. Maximal assistance to gather ADL supplies.
6. Dynamic sitting and standing balance are fair; static sitting and standing balance are fair to good.
7. Minimal assistance with transfers because of his balance deficit and poor safety awareness.
8. Minimal to moderate assistance to ambulate with a hemi-walker. Thomas is able to bear weight on the left leg, however has difficulty with shifting weight to the left side.
9. Minimal assistance with wheelchair mobility to avoid hitting objects on the left side.
10. Dependent with simple meal preparation activities. When ambulating in the kitchen with the hemi-walker and assistance, he needed cues to find the silverware drawer and the cereal cabinet (he previously was independent in getting himself breakfast).
11. Dependent in yard work.
12. Dependent in handling family finances. Thomas was unable to fill out a check correctly to pay the electric bill.

Thomas is right hand dominant. A/PROM, strength and endurance in his right upper extremity is WNL. Grip and pinch strength in his right hand are WNL. Sensation is intact in his RUE. His RUE is functional.

Thomas's LUE is nonfunctional. His LUE is painful and hypersensitive to touch. His left hand is moderately to severely edematous and hot to touch. There are P/AROM limitations in finger flexion. There are also P/AROM limitations in his left shoulder as well as a one finger breadth subluxation. He tends to cradle his arm close to his body and doesn't want anyone to touch it.

The following PROM limitations are noted in his LUE secondary to pain and hypertonicity: Left shoulder flexion (0 to 110); left shoulder abduction (0 to 90); and left external rotation (0 to 20). Thomas has moderate hypertonicity in left scapular retractors and depressors, shoulder extensors and adductors, and mild hypertonicity in elbow flexors, forearm pronators, wrist and finger flexors. All other muscle groups are hypotonic. He demonstrates partial motion in all joints in both flexor and extensor patterns. Sensation for proprioception, light touch, and stereognosis are moderately impaired in the LUE.

Thomas was admitted to your rehabilitation hospital on June 9th where the average length of stay for a client post CVA is 3 to 4 weeks. Discharge plans are to send Thomas home. Thomas' wife states that she will be able to care for him. What will you do to help Thomas?

In order to use a client-centered approach, select one person in your group to "be" Thomas. This person can then tell you about his roles, tasks, activities, interests, and priorities to assist you in developing your treatment plan and selecting appropriate therapeutic activities.

TUTORIAL SESSION SHEET

Case Study (Pt. Name, Dx.): *Thomas; Left Hemiplegia*

Group Members' Names: _____

Facts/Knowledge	Learning Issues	Actions/Steps to Learn
What do you already know that will help you to approach this case?	What questions do you need to ask to learn about:	What are the plans to find the answers to your questions?
1. Individual client—roles, tasks, activities	1. Individual client—roles, tasks, activities	
2. The client's physical/sociocultural environment	2. The client's physical/sociocultural environment	
3. Clinical signs and symptoms, treatment for diagnosis	3. Clinical signs and symptoms, treatment for diagnosis	

CASE STUDY TREATMENT PLAN SHEET

Case Study (Client Name; Dx.): Thomas; Left Hemiplegia

Group Members' Names: _____

Deficits	Stage-Specific Cause	Short-Term Goals	Relates to which deficit	Functional Outcomes	Relates to which STG

CASE STUDY TREATMENT PLAN SHEET

Page 2

Case Study (Client Name; Dx.): *Thomas; Left Hemiplegia*

Group Members' Names: _____

Short-Term Goals	Methods	Rationale	Tx Approach/ Frame of Reference	Specific Activity/ Modality

33

Dom

Retired Fireman with Left Hemiparesis

Dom was referred to home health OT on May 24th. The information given to you, his home health OT, is as follows:

Diagnosis: CVA; history of hypertension, coronary bypass on 5/1 (this year). He suffered a CVA during the surgery. Dom is 56 years old. He lives with his wife of 30 years in a first floor condominium on Miami Beach. His primary residence is in New York, but he lives in Florida during the winter months. He is on disability from the New York City Fire Department due to cardiac problems and a previous CVA 3 years ago. This CVA also affected his left side. Dom was unable to pass the rigorous physical tests required of NYFD firemen. He was independent in his self-care and still able to drive. Strength in his LUE was in good range, however, gross and fine motor coordination were impaired. He had limited endurance secondary to the CVA and cardiac problems.

You evaluate Dom on your first visit and find the following:

He is alert, pleasant and cooperative. He is oriented to person and place, but not to time. His long-term memory is intact, and short-term memory is impaired. Dom follows most simple commands. He is able to attend for a full therapy session (50 minutes). He has a left visual field cut and left side inattention.

Dom requires supervision with all functional transfers with the exception of shower transfers for which he requires minimal assistance. He has good sitting balance and fair dynamic standing balance. He requires contact guard assistance when ambulating with a quad cane.

Dom is right hand dominant. His RUE is functional although he complains of occasional pain in his right shoulder. He says it is arthritis due to the wear and tear of carrying heavy hoses. He attempts to use his LUE for light ADL, however, not always with success or efficiency. This frustrates him. He demonstrates isolated movement in all joints in his LUE but quickly goes into a pattern movement when moving against resistance. Gross and fine motor coordination is poor. Sensation in his LUE is mildly impaired for light touch, superficial pain, and stereognosis.

Presently, Dom needs minimal assistance with donning and doffing clothes and assistance to manage all clothes closures (i.e., buttons, zippers, snaps, shoelaces). He requires minimal assistance to bathe himself. Using an electric razor, he requires reminders to attend to the left side of his face when shaving. He requires minimal assistance to brush his teeth and to comb his hair. Dom is able to feed himself when his food is cut up for him. Dom used to help with the cooking but does none of this anymore. He especially enjoyed making homemade pasta and different types of homemade bread. He also enjoyed collecting fire department patches and building and flying model airplanes. He would like to get back to these activities. What will you do to help Dom?

In order to use a client-centered approach, select one person in your group to "be" Dom. This person can then tell you about his roles, tasks, activities, interests, and priorities (this can be "pretend") to assist you in developing your treatment plan and selecting appropriate therapeutic activities.

TUTORIAL SESSION SHEET

Case Study (Pt. Name, Dx.): Dom; Left Hemiparesis

Group Members' Names: _____

Facts/Knowledge	Learning Issues	Actions/Steps to Learn
What do you already know that will help you to approach this case?	What questions do you need to ask to learn about:	What are the plans to find the answers to your questions?
1. Individual client—roles, tasks, activities	1. Individual client—roles, tasks, activities	
2. The client's physical/sociocultural environment	2. The client's physical/sociocultural environment	
3. Clinical signs and symptoms, treatment for diagnosis	3. Clinical signs and symptoms, treatment for diagnosis	

CASE STUDY TREATMENT PLAN SHEET

Page 1

Case Study (Client Name; Dx.): Dom; Left Hemiparesis

Group Members' Names: _____

Deficits	Stage-Specific Cause	Short-Term Goals	Relates to which deficit	Functional Outcomes	Relates to which STG

CASE STUDY TREATMENT PLAN SHEET

Case Study (Client Name; Dx.): Dom; Left Hemiparesis

Group Members' Names: _____

Short-Term Goals	Methods	Rationale	Tx Approach/ Frame of Reference	Specific Activity/ Modality

34

Chapter

Martha

Homemaker with Right Hemiplegia

Martha is a 78-year-old female who was admitted to the hospital on May 21st after having suffered a CVA. On May 20th, Martha was eating a pretzel when she suddenly started choking and developed slight weakness on her right side. Her husband took her to the hospital where she was diagnosed with a transient ischemic attack (TIA). The following day Martha suffered a CVA with resultant right hemiplegia and aphasia. It is uncertain whether the client developed the CVA symptoms after the choking episode or whether the choking episode was caused by the stroke in progress (the most likely).

Martha is a homemaker and never worked outside the home. She graduated from high school. She enjoys bingo, playing solitaire and bridge, and working in her flower garden. Martha's spouse is a healthy 80-year-old. Her husband is very supportive. He states that he wants to care for her at home and will hire private assistance if he needs to. Financially he is able to do so. They have one daughter who lives in New York.

Martha is unable to express herself verbally. She is able to reliably answer yes/no questions using head nodding and shaking. Martha is alert and oriented to herself (name and birth date) but has mildly impaired orientation to time and place. Martha has a flat affect. She is able to follow simple one-step commands and can attend therapy for approximately 10 minutes with occasional redirection to the task. Martha wears eyeglasses for farsightedness (per husband). She is able to track a moving object in all fields.

Martha's static sitting balance is fair, her dynamic sitting balance and static standing balance are poor. She is unable to ambulate at this time. She requires maximal assistance with bed mobility and is dependent in wheelchair mobility. She requires maximal assistance with sit to stand transfers from the bed, mat, and chair and maximal assistance with w/c to bed and w/c to bedside

commode transfers. She has a motor planning deficit, her endurance is poor, and she has poor safety awareness.

Martha requires moderate to maximal assistance with upper body dressing and maximal assistance with lower body dressing. She is unable to gather any ADL supplies. She requires moderate assistance with brushing dentures, and maximal assistance with lower body bathing and with toilet hygiene. She requires minimal assistance to comb her hair and moderate assistance for upper body bathing. At the present time she is not having difficulty with swallowing, however she is having difficulty manipulating eating utensils with her non-dominant left hand. She is dependent in all homemaking activities.

Martha is right hand dominant. PROM in the RUE is within functional limits (WFL). She has moderate edema in the right hand and a one finger subluxation of the right shoulder. All muscle groups are hypotonic throughout. She demonstrates minimal movement at the scapula and shoulder. Her RUE is nonfunctional.

Martha has a history of a fracture of the left humerus 8 years ago. P/AROM limitations in left shoulder flexion (0 to 110), shoulder abduction (0 to 105), and external rotation (0 to 35). Strength is WFL within ROM limitations. Grip and pinch strength in the left hand are WFL. She uses her LUE for most ADL. Therapist is unable to accurately assess sensation secondary to communication deficit. It appears that sensation is intact in the LUE and impaired in the RUE (light touch, superficial pain, proprioception).

She has impaired right/left discrimination, a mild motor planning deficit, constructional apraxia, and right side inattention as noted when eating.

Martha has been admitted to your rehabilitation hospital on June 9th, where the average length of stay for a client post CVA is 3 to 4 weeks. Martha's husband is devoted to his wife and plans to bring her home after she is through with therapy. What will you do to help Martha?

Since Martha is unable to communicate—to use a client-centered approach—select one person in your group to "be" Martha's husband. This person can then tell you about Martha's roles, tasks, activities, interests, and priorities to assist you in developing your treatment plan and selecting appropriate therapeutic activities.

TUTORIAL SESSION SHEET

Case Study (Pt. Name, Dx.): Martha; Right Hemiplegia

Group Members' Names: _____

Facts/Knowledge

What do you already know that will help you to approach this case?

1. Individual client—roles, tasks, activities
2. The client's physical/sociocultural environment
3. Clinical signs and symptoms, treatment for diagnosis

Learning Issues

What questions do you need to ask to learn about:

1. Individual client—roles, tasks, activities
2. The client's physical/sociocultural environment
3. Clinical signs and symptoms, treatment for diagnosis

Actions/Steps to Learn

What are the plans to find the answers to your questions?

CASE STUDY TREATMENT PLAN SHEET

Page 1

Case Study (Client Name; Dx.): Martha; Right Hemiplegia

Group Members' Names: _____

Deficits	Stage-Specific Cause	Short-Term Goals	Relates to which deficit	Functional Outcomes	Relates to which STG

CASE STUDY TREATMENT PLAN SHEET

Page 2

Case Study (Client Name; Dx.): *Martha; Right Hemiplegia*

Group Members' Names: _____

Short-Term Goals	Methods	Rationale	Tx Approach/ Frame of Reference	Specific Activity/ Modality

35

Hank

Roofer with Traumatic Brain Injury

Hank is a 25-year-old male who is employed as a roofer. He is single and still lives with his parents in a townhouse. Hank graduated from high school (barely) and immediately began working at his present job. He enjoys hanging out at singles bars, attending football games, watching sci-fi movies on TV, and riding his Harley. On November 10th he suffered a traumatic brain injury in a fall from the roof of a one story house. His employer states that he was not surprised because Hank tended to be accident prone. Hank was admitted to your rehabilitation hospital on November 22nd.

In reviewing the medical chart, you find out that Hank was in a coma for a week in the acute care hospital. He received OT at the acute care hospital which consisted of sensory stimulation first, then cognitive retraining and neuromuscular developmental therapy after he emerged from the coma. The social worker states in her notes that the discharge plan is for Hank to return home to live with his parents and to attend the sheltered workshop near his home, a 10 minute bus ride away. At the present time both his parents have full-time jobs. His mother described Hank as being a "mama's boy" and being very dependent in home-making chores such as cooking, cleaning, and washing clothes. His mother also stated that Hank took care of his own finances and his checking account. He paid rent to live at home.

You see Hank for the first time on November 27th. Hank is pleasant and alert. You note that his left eye deviates inward. Hank is able to follow simple commands but his processing time and response time is slow. He knows his name and can give personal information about himself. He is able to tell you where he lives, the name of the acute care hospital where he was, and the name of the rehabilitation hospital. He needs minimal verbal cueing to remember the date and the time of day. He has poor concept of passage of time as he thinks he was only in the rehabilitation hospital for a few hours. He requires moderate cueing to follow his daily schedule. He also has poor topographical orientation. He frequently gets lost and cannot find his room on the rehabilitation wing.

Hank has a mild short-term memory deficit. His long-term memory is good. He remembers incidents up to 5 minutes before his fall from the roof. He remembers "waking up" to find his mother at his bedside reading a book to him. His concentration is poor and his attention span is poor. He needs frequent redirection to tasks. He has poor problem-solving ability, he lacks insight into his disabilities, he demonstrates poor safety awareness, and he is impulsive. He is unable to do simple math calculations.

Hank experiences diplopia, which interferes with his reading. If he closes his left eye, he is able to track an object in all planes with his right eye. He also has a mild figure ground deficit.

Hank is right hand dominant. His RUE is functional. He demonstrates ataxic like movements and dysmetria in his LUE. He demonstrates isolated control, and muscle strength is fair throughout his LUE. Muscle tone is hypotonic throughout the left upper extremity. Proprioception and kinesthesia are mildly impaired in the LUE. Sensation for light touch and superficial pain are intact. Fine and gross motor coordination in the LUE are poor. He uses his LUE as an active stabilizer for tasks close to his body.

His static sitting balance is good. His dynamic sitting balance is fair to good. He is able to ambulate, however he does so tentatively with a wide base. He is able to get in and out of bed independently. He is able to transfer sit to stand from the bed independently. He needs supervision to contact guard assist to transfer to and from a regular toilet and in and out of the bathtub. Hank requires minimal assistance with upper and lower body dressing due to decreased functional use of his LUE, balance problems, and difficulty attending to and sequencing the tasks. He is able to shave with an electric razor, brush his teeth, and to comb his hair when the items are prepared for him. He is able to feed himself with his dominant right hand if his food is prepared and cut for him.

Hank is very anxious to return home and resume his normal leisure activities but he is concerned about returning to work. He tells you that his lawyer has told him they are seeking a million dollar settlement for damages resulting from the fall. He tells you he plans to use this money to buy a horse farm in North Georgia. He tells you he will be "sitting pretty" with this million bucks, won't have to work and doesn't want to.

What will you do to help Hank?

In order to use a client-centered approach, select one person in your group to "be" Hank. This person can then tell you about his roles, tasks, activities, interests, and priorities to assist you in developing your treatment plan and selecting appropriate therapeutic activities.

TUTORIAL SESSION SHEET

Case Study (Pt. Name, Dx.): Hank; Traumatic Brain Injury

Group Members' Names: _____

Facts/Knowledge

What do you already know that will help you to approach this case?

1. Individual client—roles, tasks, activities
2. The client's physical/sociocultural environment
3. Clinical signs and symptoms, treatment for diagnosis

Learning Issues

What questions do you need to ask to learn about:

1. Individual client—roles, tasks, activities
2. The client's physical/sociocultural environment
3. Clinical signs and symptoms, treatment for diagnosis

Actions/Steps to Learn

What are the plans to find the answers to your questions?

CASE STUDY TREATMENT PLAN SHEET

Case Study (Client Name; Dx.): Hank; Traumatic Brain Injury

Group Members' Names: _____

Deficits	Stage-Specific Cause	Short-Term Goals	Relates to which deficit	Functional Outcomes	Relates to which STG

CASE STUDY TREATMENT PLAN SHEET

Page 2

Case Study (Client Name; Dx.): Hank; *Traumatic Brain Injury*

Group Members' Names: _____

Short-Term Goals	Methods	Rationale	Tx Approach/ Frame of Reference	Specific Activity/ Modality

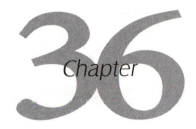

Bill

Unskilled Worker with Traumatic Brain Injury

Bill, 22 years old, is admitted to your rehabilitation facility s/p traumatic brain injury suffered in an automobile accident. Bill was drinking with some friends at the Beer House when he was challenged to a drag race. During the race he lost control of his automobile. It rolled over two times. Miraculously he suffered no broken bones, however he did have some minor lacerations and his head hit the windshield because he wasn't wearing a seat belt.

Bill dropped out of school when he was 16 years old. Bill's parents have been to visit once. Bill and his parents are not on good terms. His mother states that he was a difficult child and they were happy to see him move out. At the time of the accident, Bill was living with a girlfriend whom he met 4 months ago. She was supporting him. The girlfriend left town to visit friends on the other coast. It is expected that she will be gone for about a month. Bill, although presently unemployed, has held several low paying jobs, the longest for 7 months. Bill's brother states that Bill gets "tired" of a job and just doesn't go back. Bill's brother visits every day but does not want to be responsible for him.

Bill is not oriented to time, place, or person. Bill has not recognized any of his family members. He has short-term memory deficit and limited attention span. Bill has no recollection of his accident or the events leading to it.

Bill is easily distracted in the clinic and refuses to participate in therapy. Bill is agitated and frequently becomes verbally and physically abusive to staff and clients. He has difficulty with simple tasks such as getting dressed. He is not able to use eating utensils appropriately. This frustrates him and agitates him further.

Bill is able to ambulate without an assistive device. Muscle tone, control, and strength are WFL in all extremities. Since his admission 4 days ago, he has tried to walk out of the hospital eight times. When attempting to leave the facility, Bill insists the staff needs to let him go to get to his job with the "CIA." He frequently wanders from his room at night, requiring the night nurses to supervise him closely.

What will you do to help Bill?

In order to use a client-centered approach, select one person in your group to "be" Bill. This person can then tell you about his roles, tasks, activities, interests, and priorities to assist you in developing your treatment plan and selecting appropriate therapeutic activities.

TUTORIAL SESSION SHEET

Case Study (Pt. Name, Dx.): Bill; Traumatic Brain Injury

Group Members' Names: _____

Facts/Knowledge	Learning Issues	Actions/Steps to Learn
What do you already know that will help you to approach this case? 1. Individual client—roles, tasks, activities 2. The client's physical/sociocultural environment 3. Clinical signs and symptoms, treatment for diagnosis	What questions do you need to ask to learn about: 1. Individual client—roles, tasks, activities 2. The client's physical/sociocultural environment 3. Clinical signs and symptoms, treatment for diagnosis	What are the plans to find the answers to your questions?

Case Study Treatment Plan Sheet

Case Study (Client Name; Dx.): Bill; Traumatic Brain Injury

Group Members' Names: _____

Page 1

Deficits	Stage-Specific Cause	Short-Term Goals	Relates to which deficit	Functional Outcomes	Relates to which STG

Case Study Treatment Plan Sheet

Case Study (Client Name; Dx.): Bill; Traumatic Brain Injury

Group Members' Names: _____

Short-Term Goals	Methods	Rationale	Tx Approach/ Frame of Reference	Specific Activity/ Modality

37

Chapter

Van

Accounts Manager with Brain Injury

Van, 45 years old, suffered a severe head injury in a skiing accident when he went off the trail and ran into a tree. He is admitted to your rehabilitation hospital 3 weeks later. Van is posturing in a decorticate posture with his UE in shoulders adducted, internally rotated, elbows flexed, forearms pronated, and wrist and fingers flexed. Severe hypertonicity is present in the scapula and shoulder muscle groups, elbow flexors, forearm pronators, wrist and finger flexors limiting PROM. His LEs are positioned in extension, adduction and internal rotation with severe hypertonicity present in these muscle groups. Grasp reflexes are present in both hands.

Van responds with a groan to vigorous shaking and a loud voice with a groan and has very limited movement in all four extremities. When pressure is applied over the nail bed of one of his little fingers, he responds with eye opening, makes an unintelligible sound, and his UEs move further into flexion.

Van has a high pressure job with Smith Blarney, a financial firm. He manages several large accounts. He enjoyed his leisure time and spent much of that time at his mountain cabin with his wife and his dog, Misha. At the cabin he spent time cross-country skiing, chopping wood for his wood stove, and making wood furniture. His wife and two teenage children are very supportive and are anxious for Van to recover. You are the OT working with the rehabilitation team. What will you do to help Van and his family?

In order to use a client-centered approach, select one person in your group to "be" Van's wife. This person can then tell you about Van's roles, tasks, activities, interests, and priorities to assist you in developing your treatment plan and selecting appropriate therapeutic activities.

TUTORIAL SESSION SHEET

Case Study (Pt. Name, Dx.): Van; Brain Injury

Group Members' Names: _____

Facts/Knowledge

What do you already know that will help you to approach this case?

1. Individual client—roles, tasks, activities
2. The client's physical/sociocultural environment
3. Clinical signs and symptoms, treatment for diagnosis

Learning Issues

What questions do you need to ask to learn about:

1. Individual client—roles, tasks, activities
2. The client's physical/sociocultural environment
3. Clinical signs and symptoms, treatment for diagnosis

Actions/Steps to Learn

What are the plans to find the answers to your questions?

CASE STUDY TREATMENT PLAN SHEET

Case Study (Client Name; Dx.): Van; Brain Injury

Group Members' Names: _____

Page 1

Deficits	Stage-Specific Cause	Short-Term Goals	Relates to which deficit	Functional Outcomes	Relates to which STG

Case Study Treatment Plan Sheet

Case Study (Client Name; Dx.): *Van; Brain Injury*

Group Members' Names: _____

Short-Term Goals	Methods	Rationale	Tx Approach/ Frame of Reference	Specific Activity/ Modality

Bibliography

Barrows, H. S. (1994). *Practice-based learning: Problem-based learning applied to medical education.* Springfield, IL: Southern Illinois University School of Medicine.

Barrows, H. S., & MacRae, H. (1992). *The tutorial process in problem-based learning* [Videorecording]. Springfield, IL: Southern Illinois University School of Medicine.

Borcherding, S. (2000). *Documentation manual for writing SOAP notes in occupational therapy.* Thorofare, NJ: SLACK Incorporated.

Borg, B., & Bruce, M. A. G. (1991). *The group system: the therapeutic activity group in occupational therapy.* Thorofare, NJ: SLACK Incorporated.

Fleming, M. (1991). The therapist with the three-track mind. *Am J Occup Ther, 45(8),* 1007-1014.

Hay, J. A. (1995). Investigating the development of self-evaluation skills in a problem-based tutorial course. *Acad Med, 70(8),* 733-735.

Hill, W. F. (1977). *Learning through discussion: guide for leaders and members of discussion groups.* Beverly Hills, CA: Sage Publications, Inc.

Law, M., Polatajko, H., Baptiste, S., & Townsend, E. (1997). Core concepts of occupational therapy. In E. Townsend (Ed.). *Enabling occupation: An occupational therapy perspective* (p. 29-56). Ottawa, Ontario: CAOT Publications ACE.

Mattingly, C., & Fleming, M. H. (1994). *Clinical reasoning: forms of inquiry in a therapeutic practice.* Philadelphia, PA: F. A. Davis Company.

Mosey, A. C. (1976). *Activities therapy.* New York, NY: Raven Press, Publishers.

Neistadt, M. E. (1998). Teaching clinical reasoning as a thinking frame. *Am J Occup Ther, 52(3),* 221-229.

Neistadt, M. E., Wight, J., & Mulligan, S. E. (1998). Clinical reasoning case studies as teaching tools. *Am J Occup Ther, 52(2)* 125-132.

Index of Cases

Index

BUILD *Your Library*

This book and many others on numerous different topics are available from SLACK Incorporated. For further information or a copy of our latest catalog, contact us at:

Professional Book Division
SLACK Incorporated
6900 Grove Road
Thorofare, NJ 08086 USA
Telephone: 1-856-848-1000
1-800-257-8290
Fax: 1-856-853-5991
E-mail: orders@slackinc.com
www.slackbooks.com

We accept most major credit cards and checks or money orders in US dollars drawn on a US bank. Most orders are shipped within 72 hours.

Contact us for information on recent releases, forthcoming titles, and bestsellers. If you have a comment about this title or see a need for a new book, direct your correspondence to the Editorial Director at the above address.

Thank you for your interest and we hope you found this work beneficial.